PRAISE FOR
HEALING JOURNEYS
THROUGH THE ART OF JIN SHIN JYUTSU

"Through her career as a Jin Shin Jyutsu practitioner, Nicole has touched and transformed many lives. Every story is filled with heart warming moments how Nicole has healed patients from all walks of lives and restore the balance and vitality of their health. The art of Jin Shin Jyutsu is profound and mind-blowing. I hope this book will eventually raise the awareness of this alternative healing therapy and inspire more people to join Nicole in learning this little-known but powerful method of energy healing."

David Goh
3rd Generation Master
www.imperialharvest.com

"Whether you end up as a believer or disbeliever, this book serves certainly to inspire and give hope (maybe a tear too) with each story coming to life and the full book taking us through the lens of the author's life journey. Above all we discover that success depends not only on the skill of the JSJ practitioner, but on the patient's ability to deploy "open mind and will" and "conscious practice discipline. Great first book, Nicole! Thanks for sharing!"

Joseph Francis
Adviser to Start-up Enterprise

"This book is unique and brilliant. With a deep knowledge and understanding of Jin Shin Jyutsu, Nicole presented compelling evidence of this healing art based on her clients' experience. I would gift this book to anyone who is curious to know more about JSJ and its potential for transformative healing."

Angela Tan
Founder and Life Coach, Universal Arts Pte Ltd

"Very insightful with all the various real life experiences that have been shared along with personal insights. And yet it has been written in a manner such that is easy to comprehend as well as engaging to the reader. I would definitely recommend this awesome book to anyone seeking complementary healing methods without any side effects. Wonderful Works!"

Luxshmi Bhat
Translator

"This collection of stories from Nicole is written with much love, sincerity and care. Through honest and vulnerable sharing of the journey that began with her daughter's anxiety and closed with how she managed to recover for Bell's Palsy, Nicole offers hope to all who are open to this alternative pathway to recovery. It is clear through the collection of stories in the book that when one is open, willing and committed enough in engaging in the practice of JSJ, it is possible to achieve harmony in body, mind and spirit. This is a book that is needed to demonstrate how science and art can coexist and Nicole is in a unique position to share it as she is both a psychologist and a practitioner of JSJ."

Winifred Ling
Couples Therapist/Relationship Coach/
Positive Psychology Practitioner.

PRAISE FOR NICOLE'S WORK

With Nicole's 'light touches' I felt my body responding and there seemed to be some healing. JSJ helped to ease my pain during that period of time and has contributed to my well-being. I was so relieved and truly believed God had sent me an Angel to look after me during the trying time I was going through. I am convinced that the 'power of touch' through JSJ works.

—*Jayanthi K, Cancer survivor*

✳ ✳ ✳

The tightness and keloid in my breast and leg which bothered me for the past 8 months...gone!

—*YS, CEO of an insurance company,*
2nd time Cancer Survivor.

✳ ✳ ✳

I have headache, stomach bloatedness, indigestion, constipation, numbness in fingers, aches and pain, insomnia, fatigue, low energy... after going through chemo! Amazingly, after the first session with Nicole, I continue to feel energy flowing in both my hands and that persistent blood-stained rashes had disappeared! I continued to release a lot of 'smelly gas' over the next few days. Overall, I feel energised and calm after each session.

—*SL Teo, Cancer Survivor*

✳ ✳ ✳

As my autoimmune illness increases the chances of lymphoma, I decided to restart JSJ with Nicole and practice the self-help flows that Nicole taught me. In July, my blood test results were surprisingly better than I had hoped for. My LDH dropped from 296 to 180 (normal). I am sure JSJ contributed positively to the better than expected results.

—Ms B Teoh, homemaker

✳ ✳ ✳

I was diagnosed with hyperthyroid when I came to see Nicole. Over a course of 6 sessions, my conditions (e.g. feeling flushed) were stabilised and I was off my thyroid medication earlier than other patients. Today, I continue my JSJ sessions with Nicole, maintaining my general wellbeing and self-care. Nicole is highly intuitive and experienced. With her support, JSJ has transformed my life positively in a gentle and powerful way. I highly recommend JSJ with Nicole.

—Angela Tan, Founder and Life Coach, Universal Arts Pte Ltd

✳ ✳ ✳

I have a rare illness and have gone through 2 brain bypass surgeries. I usually feel a deeper sense of rest after the JSJ session. I will highly recommend Nicole as she is competent and passionate about the work that she does to help others through self-healing. Thanks Nicole!

—Winifred Ling, Private Counselling Psychologist,
Promises Healthcare

✳ ✳ ✳

I have a medical history of respiratory issues. During the JSJ session, my body experienced deep relaxation. My airways seem to open up and felt less restrictive and my wheezing sound subsided. My initial short shallow breaths amazingly became long deep breaths and my entire being was at ease over time and I fell into deep sleep. Post session, my dry irritating throat and cough had disappeared! I did not need inhaler nor medication. Thank you JSJ for saving me from any virus or prevention from developing into acute pneumonia.

—Mr SJI, Advisor to Start-up Enterprise

✳ ✳ ✳

My aunty Catherine had a stroke in late Sep 2020. Her movements were fine but she lost her short term memory. Before she started JSJ, she would often say she didn't know what was happening to her. She forgot how to send WhatsApp messages, check her email. The left side of her face was somewhat droopy. After 6 weeks of therapy, Aunty has improved vastly. She no longer says she doesn't know what is happening to her. She's able to send out clear messages on her phone, and she's very aware of herself. The left side of her face is less droopy and she can even wink with both eyes. She has been doing her homework by holding her fingers. Thank you Nicole!

—Aunty Catherine's niece, Hui Min

✳ ✳ ✳

I asked for medication from my son who is a doctor to treat my pain. Instead, he strongly recommended that I see Nicole for therapy. In one session, not only Nicole had helped me feel better, the stiffness and pain I have been bearing in my right sole was completely gone! My legs and joints felt lighter and my movement was much smoother and without pain now! I am glad that this light touch therapy help me.

—Mrs LYeo, retired teacher

✳ ✳ ✳

After your session with AnnaB (*special needs*), she is indeed visibly in a brighter mood, happier and feels 'lighter'. Many, many thanks for helping me out with AnnaB. You came at a time when I was desperate.

—*Tania, Mother*

✳ ✳ ✳

My daughter actually becomes less stressed after the session.

—*MC, Mother of 10 yr-old girl*

The one session of JSJ with Nicole today not only improved my vision clarity, the intense itch in my eyes are completely and I do not have to put any eye drops! In addition, the blockages and tension which I have been suffering at the back of my head also eased up and disappeared after the session. Thank you for the JSJ session!

—*Yi Wei, Founder of the Conscious Studio*

✳ ✳ ✳

My mum has suffered insomnia for many months. She could hardly sleep at night and has to depend on medicine in order to sleep. After each treatment, not only was she more relaxed, she could sleep even longer hours and gradually back to her normal sleep cycle, without medication. We are all glad to see her recovery. Grateful to Nicole for her patience and guidance.

—*Lilian, private nurse*

✳ ✳ ✳

Honestly I can't even begin to describe how good I feel every time I have a JSJ session with Nicole. It's like I'm almost fighting my insomnia. I always feel like something profoundly good has changed in my body's energy at the very least. I admire what you do, so much. I truly feel that what you're doing is godsend.

—*Marcus, Psychology Undergraduate*

* * *

Given my insomniac nature, I would normally be very groggy when I got up, not feeling good at all, exhausted or feeling anxious. This was nothing like either of those. The transition between sleep to awake to sleep was incredibly smooth. My body definitely felt lighter. Emotionally, it was probably the most immensely soothing and calming feel I've experienced in a long time!

—*Mr MChiang, Executive in Healthcare Service*

* * *

I sought out Nicole's help to aid me in my most challenging period of life; I lost my dear dad and moved out alone. JSJ is extremely effective as a kickstarter for energy. I feel warmth in my veins and better energy. I also find the self-help poses Nicole shared very useful to practise on a daily basis. Personally, I would recommend jsj to anyone who wants to heal their emotions through bodywork. I find jsj touches through Nicole – comforting and non-intrusive. I find that Nicole cares for her clients and is a very experienced therapist in this field. Thank you, Nicole!

—*Kasandra, Professional services*

Healing Journeys Through The Art of Jin Shin Jyutsu

A heart warming collection of hope and self care

Nicole Ting

Photography:Simon Berger

Edited by Jayanthi Kanagaratnam

Model: Melanie GM

DEDICATION

In loving memories of Master Jiro Murai and his two main entrusted disciples Mary Burmeister and Dr Haruki Kato.

CONTENT

CHAPTER 1

Why this book?

Do you believe that each of us have this innate healing potential and power within us? Do you believe that our hands have the healing power to jump start ourselves when our life force is depleted? Have you ever experienced in your younger days a small cut on your finger and not care much about it and yet it heals pretty fast and well without much scar? Have you also noticed in your later years a similar small cut on your finger may not necessarily have the same speed of recovery and for some, the scarring remains?

I am often intrigued how our body responds to stimuli (external or internal) and how we as living organisms are capable of living a harmonious and stress-free life despite all the challenges in our lifetime.

To be honest, it took me decades to summon enough courage to write this book. It never crossed my mind that I would be so blessed to witness so many amazing healing journeys with this magnificent Art of Jin Shin Jyutsu! Over these 15 years since I learnt about JSJ, I am humbly blessed to experience personally and witnessed the limitless benefits through Jin Shin Jyutsu therapy on my clients. The conviction to share with the world about this amazing Art eventually overshadows my own insecurity and fear of being laughed at for sharing *INCREDIBLE* accounts.

The short compilation of heart rendering recounts of each healing journey is dedicated to the following groups of people:

- Those who are exhausted with being prescribed multiple drugs due to their ongoing struggles with bodily 'malfunctions'.

- Those who are literally fighting against 'mysterious and big medical labels'.
- Those who are open to alternative healing therapies that complement whatever state they are currently experiencing.
- Those who are dealing with mental-emotional challenges.
- Those who are caregivers of special needs, sick or aged persons round the clock.
- Everyone who is new in the Jin Shin Jyutsu community.

My main desire of penning these experiences is that I hope to reach out to everyone through the different healing accounts. May the sharings inspire and empower all of us to take positive actions to do something good for ourselves as we DO have this innate power of self healing. May it also give HOPE to all who are in the midst of challenging circumstances. Hang in there!

CHAPTER 2

What is Jin Shin Jyutsu?

The art of Jin Shin Jyutsu hails from an ancient oriental origin of more than 3000 years. It is an ancient art of healing which involves harmonising the energy system within the body.

It is based on the principle that our body has many energy channels that nourishes every cell within every organ of our body and regulates their functioning. When one or more of these channels are disrupted due to a variety of reasons (external and internal stressors such as emotional disturbances; mental anxieties and worries; lifestyle diet; physical strains and injuries etc.) the energy flow is blocked. These blockages may lead to unpleasant symptoms and dis-eases.

Jin Shin Jyutsu (JSJ) therapy is a safe and non-invasive way of balancing this life energy within us. Through gentle placing of our hands on different key areas of the body, we can bring about a harmonious outcome for ourselves and others. Unlike other treatments which either sedates or stimulates, JSJ harmonises our life energy, through gentle touch, allowing our internal adjustment to happen entirely on its own. Hence, it is a great way to facilitate the body to return to its harmonious state physically and emotionally. Not only does it promote one's inherent ability to heal, it serves as a valuable **complement** to conventional healing methods for all ages. It is also important to note that it does not replace the advice of your own physician or other healthcare professionals.

Jin Shin Jyutsu was rediscovered by Master Jiro Murai in Japan in 1912, after he had healed himself from a life-threatening illness. To promote the development of the Art of Jin Shin Jyutsu for future generations, Master Jiro Murai devoted the rest of his life to the research on this Art that included studying and interpreting the Kojiki ("Record of Ancient Things") in the Japanese Imperial Archives.

Thankfully, the Art of Jin Shin Jyutsu was passed down to Mary Burmeister, one of his entrusted students, a first generation Japanese American, who went to Japan in the late 1940s. In the 1950s, Mary brought this Art of Jin Shin Jyutsu to the United States and as a result of her effort, Jin Shin Jyutsu Scottsdale was established as the headquarter for all official Jin Shin Jyutsu workshops. This awesome Art is now practised worldwide in many countries and has many thousands of students as well as practitioners worldwide.

For more information about Jin Shin Jyutsu and classes worldwide, do visit the websites www.jsjinc.net and jinshininstitute.com

CHAPTER 3

How I stumbled upon JSJ?

Background

I had the first "glimpse" of JSJ during a chance meeting with Angie, a mother with an autistic child in a special school. That was in 1998. I was a practising psychologist in a special school then. Never did I expect that this chance meeting with Angie would turn out to be a pivotal point in my life ...

Her child, then aged seven, was diagnosed by the school's senior psychologist with severe autism and the form-teacher of his class found it extremely difficult to manage him. He was observed to display numerous challenging kinds of behaviour and in socially inappropriate ways. Very often he would refuse or ignore requests and do the exact opposite of what the teacher would ask of him. Due to his high sensory sensitivities, he would often seek out various stimulation through his touch, smell and even sound. Every day, he would find something to 'engage' himself with, instead of paying attention in class. At times, he would cover both his ears because he could tune in to the birds singing outside the window of his class, or he would tune in to even higher frequency of vibrations many of us could not pick up on. Sometimes, he would run out of the classroom and when found, he would be rubbing his face against the trunk of a tree as it seemed to give him comfort and security. At other times, he would raise his hand and touch and feel the textile design of a blouse which a female teacher was wearing, not with any ill intentions. When on public transport, he had to be hand held tightly as there was the fear that he would dash out of the train without much concern for safety. Hence, the school adopted and implemented numerous behavioural management strategies to help him but without much success.

The School Management Committee hence ordered Angie to remain outside her son's classroom, for as long as he was in school. Angie had to sacrifice her time to be in school the whole day for Ken. In my opinion, her presence in school served as a 'relief' to the teachers who (unfortunately) could not manage him to the 'expectations' that the school wanted. Rain or shine, her unfailing love and perseverance prevailed. She would sit outside his classroom for hours on a daily basis to monitor him, from the start, to the end of the school day. She did that every day without fail for months. That's how our paths crossed.

Every day, when I passed by the classroom during my rounds, I would see her. She was always neatly and simply dressed and without fail, reading a book. Our initial nods to each other when we passed each other turned into smiles then greetings. These grew into meaningful conversations of sharing and discussing interesting topics of alternative therapies she had sought to help her child. Through her, I could sense how much love and sacrifice she had gone through to find a 'cure' for her child. She gave up a promising nursing career, and she put her whole life on hold to care 24/7 for her child without any complaints. Instead of giving up or accepting what traditional medical bodies advocated that her child would never be cured of ASD, she held onto the firm belief that there was always a way to 'save' him. With this *great motivating push*, she never stopped looking for a solution to assist him. Her search went far and wide. Of the many therapies and courses she picked up, she found Jin Shin Jyutsu as the *perfect* therapy for her child.

My reflection

I feel that as educators, we can often fail to see that such challenging behaviour, as we term them, as the manifestations of high sensory disharmonies. The teachers in special schools ought to have good understanding and knowledge to empathise first and then plan constructive interventions to help children like Ken to cope with his sensory, behavioural and emotional outbursts. Instead of sending children like him home as punishment (or an easy way out), appropriate follow up actions and constructive 'punishment' should be explored.

Ken was sent home frequently as the behaviour management plan seemed to often fail or rather work well, depending which perspective one takes! Sending home was the answer to eliminating misbehaviour (= Absence in class = Absence of misbehaviour = successful implementation of plans). Personally, sending a sensory loaded child home each time a teacher cannot cope is NOT the answer to solving challenging misbehaviour. It is a disaster when a special need school teacher cannot cope with dealing with a child's behaviour. Everyone has to work together to closely monitor and adapt the strategies for the best outcome for the child. In Ken's case, there was absolutely no follow up support for the family once he was sent home...for a day, then a week, and eventually months...

I often wonder when the school 'strategised' on such a level, and offered no support to the mother who had to deal with him at home, I could see the impending consequence they were heading. Unfortunately for this case, Ken was eventually 'phased' out of the school, given the frequency of the 'sending home consequence'. With no help at hand, his mother Angie hit rock bottom. She sought out different options and never stopped exploring and learning many different types of therapies in search of a cure for Ken.

All that I have narrated about Ken was when he was younger. Ken is now in his adulthood. The progress he has made since, is indeed remarkable! He has progressed from being dependent in all areas of his life to being an independent being and even contributing to society meaningfully. He is working now; he takes the public transport on his own and even helps out at home with laundry and cooking! For leisure, he plays golf with his father and even does his own JSJ self-help practice for himself. He is the **most well balanced and harmonised** ASD individual I have ever encountered in my life and work. (I am not lying!) What is even more amazing and incredible is that his state of harmony and progress is attributed to the magic of this beautiful Universal Art of Harmonising energy, Jin Shin Jyutsu. No other traditional or specialised interventions could give him a glimpse of hope or chance of recovery then.

Due to this amazing harmony brought about through the JSJ therapy, Ken' cognitive and social aspects expanded. When he was still a teen, he became interested in learning and asked to have tuition. Ken has many amazing talents. From a young age, he has enjoyed drawing and would immerse himself all day-long drawing and colouring pictures of animals. Besides Art, he is musically inclined too, as he can play a long didgeridoo, an aboriginal wind instrument which poses great difficulty for many of us to pick up and blow with such accuracy and form. Ken did this without much difficulty and quickly mastered this art. He is often mesmerised by the tones from this instrument and has found such great affinity to this magical device that brings him calmness and peace. He would spend many hours deeply entrenched in playing the instrument, like the deft hands of a gifted weaver.

I am truly amazed by the "extraordinary" progress Ken had made over the years with JSJ *alone*. He has gone beyond traditional medical treatment, as well as sidestepped cognitive cum behavioural interventions that psychology prescribed.

Very often, the sacrifice that the main caregiver makes goes unnoticed. Sometimes, it is even taken for granted. As a mother, many demands are made of us. Often such perceptions leave us feeling exhausted, helpless and suicidal.

The sacrifices that mother Angie has made is 'countless' and invisible to many of us. The endless heartaches, struggles and battles she had to put up with against all the outbursts, meltdowns and challenging milestones, to grasping onto dwindling hopes and increasing doubts and frustrations of finding that nothing works to...

tears of sadness,
tears of frustrations,
tears of loneliness,
and tears of uncertainty.

To date, this young and handsome boy has grown into an independent citizen with excellent life skills- without the help of any special school education and support – during his most needed milestones. Not only is he happily employed, he cooks, cleans and does laundry and cares for his parents!

Such unconditional and tireless love... Ken is the most fortunate and blessed child! My tribute and my utter gratitude goes to Ken and his mother for introducing and encouraging me to learn this beautiful ART of life.

Unfulfilling Psychology at work

In retrospect, I see my journey somewhat similar to Angie. We are both seekers of impactful and *real remedies*; she for Ken, I for the students I serve.

I did enjoy working with the beneficiaries of my work during my school attachment and I had an eventful journey in my career as a psychologist in the public service and special schools. However, I felt that the impact that I had made was very superficial. Besides the responsibilities of supporting more than 20 mainstream schools; spearheading and monitoring of specialised psycho-educational support programmes; the weekly school visits for case referrals, class observations, case assessments and scheduled trainings for teachers, there was also the 'pressure' of hitting the target number of assessment reports we needed to fulfil to be deemed within the 'acceptable range' of KPI performance.

Like a factory worker on a production line, many colleagues and I spent the majority of our time rushing to churn out numerous overdue psychological assessment reports from time to time. We had to meet the given target number of assessment reports per month to justify a 'higher order' agenda. We churned out assessment reports that no one would pay much real attention to. The real needs of the clients seemed to take second place. Recommendations that required intensive and face-to-face interventions were often brushed aside. This was due to the "BIGGER" reasons that needed to be considered such as constraints of resources, time and expertise. Initially, I joined in the 'madness', rushing through reports and hoping the reports would help the clients. I even wondered what the point was of chasing after certificates in attending courses and NOT being able to do the real hands-on work. What was the point of being called a psychologist in the system, only to become another specialised machine in conducting assessments and churning out assessment reports day in and day out.

Over the years, like many practising professionals, as my tool kit of 'expertise' grew into a huge tool box, I actively and hungrily sought out needy cases to work with in the special schools. Some of the programmes which I initiated included- Social skills Training, Anger Management and Psycho-cognitive training. Despite making good progress, many programmes which I started, eventually could not be sustained due to logistics and support problems.

As I continued to search for answers through the various assessment tools, techniques and courses to help my clients-students, family and teachers, I realised that there was much MORE I could do. Though I had witnessed the positive effects of conventional therapies, I became more in awe of those cases which Angie shared with me. Many had tried traditional methods but yielded little outcomes. Yet with JSJ therapy, all of them had demonstrated a deep level of harmonising and lasting outcome.

At that point of time, to embrace JSJ in my profession as a psychologist was something that never crossed my mind ...

Small Steps in My JSJ Journey and My Initial 'Guinea Pigs'

Being a realist rather than an idealist, together with my professional training and experience, (and my limited understanding of this Art), I was very cautious NOT to be fooled by this iffy concept of intervention. Well, that was how most 'mainstream' professionals would view it then now...including my naive self then! However, I could not deny that I felt drawn to JSJ and how it could be used to help the "problem" students or anyone else with various problems. As sceptical as I was, I was amazed by the "extraordinary" progress Ken had made, beyond the traditional medical as well as cognitive cum behavioural interventions that psychology brought with it.

As JSJ was a relatively new and unknown modality to this part of the world then in 1990s, before my official first 5-days class with Philomena, I met with Angie and few interested parties frequently to discuss and 'practise' 'techniques' among ourselves from the book, "The touch of healing" by Alice Burmeister and with Tom Monte.

It is my FIRST book on Jin Shin Jyutsu before I embarked on my first class with esteemed JSJ instructress Philomena Dooley. I have read and reread it so many times over the decades. Each time I read the book, I am in awe of the 'miracles'... I have never grown tired of reading it! I have not been able to keep this fire of enthusiasm to myself and have shared this therapy with my friends, colleagues and family!

Setbacks all the way

I have encountered MANY non-believers to date! I have tried over time to share my knowledge of JSJ with my community of professionals. I bought and gifted the book "The Touch of healing" to some of my colleagues hoping they too would experience its goodness. I offered to share with many teachers this amazing art of harmonising our energy systems but only faced rejection. Many are not ready to even be open to hear about this beautiful art.

I have tried to share my enthusiasm with my circle of friends but many of them shun me with the exception of Su, my best friend who is more open.

Many who are disbelievers say...

- "How can something so simple like holding fingers help at all with anything?"
- "How can such a simple act claim to be so dynamic and miraculous with just holding fingers, touching here and there to yield such over rated outcomes?"
- "So there is no need to see doctors?"

These are often the very cryptic and sarcastic replies I have had to deal with. Some disbelievers will 'veil' their so-called support through a no-show outcome when they are invited for a free talk in the earlier days.

In the earlier years of my career as a psychologist, I soon realised quite painfully that my sincerity and enthusiasm in sharing this beautiful art form seemed to bring a lot of 'cognitive dissonance' to certain people in the community; particularly those in the scientific league, many of my 'religious' peers and learned professional colleagues. At some point, it might have even 'jeopardised' or brought about a great deal of discomfort to many of them including myself, given my profession. Their response seemed to signal their disapproval and fear. Many thought that I had been 'misled' or was even out of my mind!

In the early years of my career, I worked very hard and earned good performance ranking yearly. I too thought it was important to be accepted in that community. However, it soon became clear that those sceptics and rigid learned professionals were not going to like or accept my involvement with JSJ no matter what. They had their own beliefs about what was acceptable.

I understand now that no matter how much we hear about the numerous amazing JSJ related testimonies, if we do not open our hearts to embrace it's infinite healing possibilities and decide to take that leap of faith and commitment, we can't really begin to experience for ourselves it's amazing benefits. We have to Be our own testimony. That is what I have decided to embark on.

Eventually, I gave up my futile efforts to convince that particular community that refused to even appreciate JSJ. Instead focussed my devotion into practising that Art and getting to understand it and serving those who were and are open to this alternative therapy. I hope to perhaps, be my own testimony as life goes on.

Initially I was leading a 'double' life and chose who I would share about this ART very cautiously. It put a lot of strain on me. However, over the years, the conviction to embrace JSJ 'publicly' was the next bold step. I decided to focus and pursue this Art and let go of the fear of not being part of an identified group as my conviction in JSJ grew stronger.

This is how I envisioned myself to be, that is, the first psychologist who practises the Art of Jin Shin Jyutsu in Singapore. Life events do indeed shape our decisions. Life-changing decisions are often made at the crossroad of our journey in life.

Thankfully, besides Angie, the only support I had at that point in my life was my family, husband, my two children and my BFF. They were my only "guinea pigs" then and still are my faithful subjects of JSJ practices over these years. A BIG THANK YOU for being open and trusting in the process through all the sessions we had.

As my private case referrals for JSJ therapy take flight through word of mouth over the years, I have found that JSJ fulfils my life intention – 'To be an effective tool for All who need healing In the highest form of harmony.'

Hence, my mantra is to *age with JSJ*.

I am honoured to share with you, each unique experience which JSJ has brought to my clients. I am very grateful for their consent and willingness to share their own unique struggles, pains, fears, sadness and most important of all, their evolution of their well-being and hence their exciting healing journeys.

This book is more than just a sharing of healing stories. It includes true accounts of people who have made significant changes to their health habits and reversed disharmonies that took hold of their lives. Above all, my clients and I share ONE heartfelt intention, which is to bring HOPE to whatever situation you or your family may be facing. May the book bless each reader in your search for healing in this lifetime.

CHAPTER 4

Healing Journeys

Case 1 – The start of my journey – my first 'hands flow'

My first hands-on case was my eldest daughter, Tracy during her younger days. It was through her severe panic attacks and anxiety that I came to appreciate and gain more insight and intuition about learning JSJ. I worked with her daily, to ease her condition. Being my first case, Tracy's journey was to begin my own journey of transformation with this healing art.

Severe Anxiety destroys, JSJ restores!

My eldest daughter, Tracy had an eventful birth. She was born at 38 weeks and had a challenging and stressful birth journey as the umbilicus cord was wrapped around her neck in my womb. Quite sadly, the progression of the stressful labour had partly contributed to the overall anxiety that was passed on to my baby. The late timing and amount of epidural given resulted in an overdosing effect. I could not even feel my legs, nor prop my legs up during the delivery stage. I just could not even gather my strength or feel the PUSH at all. Hence, the final stage of delivery included the vacuum extraction process. That resulted in the left side of her head being flattened for many years. Thankfully with JSJ, this has been reversed and her head is a whole round again! Upon being delivered, Tracy was a silent baby and did not cry aloud. A few days later, she developed severe jaundice and had to be hospitalised for more than a week.

As a first time mother, being traumatised with my water-bag bursting at the wee hours of the day, going into labour two weeks before the scheduled date, and then being faced with further complications, my body was under tremendous stress. My newborn too was under stress. I was not aware at all of the level of stress she had been under.

I could not breast feed her for more than one week due to the strain! To make matters worse, she could not suckle well and hence had very limited intake of breast milk. When I cuddled and carried her, instead of having a restful sleep, baby Tracy expressed her stress and tension by leaving 'biting marks' on my chest. Initially, Tracy started out with a weak constitution and would often fall ill. During those early months when Tracy fell ill so often, my initiation into 'motherhood' was really challenged!

I didn't even realise the mental and emotional stress her body had gone through during her early period of birth as I was too preoccupied with my own stress of taking care of her illness as well as handling my body undergoing tremendous changes at that period of time.

It seemed like for almost every 2 weeks, she would be afflicted with a fever, cough and phlegm. She cried a fair bit during the days and nights. To add to that, she was a very colicky baby and I was a very fatigued, frustrated and depressed new mom. Little did I realise that not only did she **not** outgrow her crying episodes, her anxiety level continued to escalate to a severely high level which further compromised her immune system.

Cumulative stress and manifestations in different areas

As she started schooling, my husband and I adopted a very 'relaxed' approach to school for our child. Despite that, Tracy exhibited school anxiety symptoms and was constantly crying before school hours. When she started primary school, every day **without** fail, at the strike of 11 a.m. when the school bus was due to arrive, the terrifying symptoms would surface. Her body would experience tremendous 'outburst of stress' as she would go into spontaneous vomiting, throwing out all the meals she had ingested. Soon she developed irritable bowel syndrome. This repulsion of food, in the form of vomit, and diarrhea would last for at least 30 minutes. This led to her losing nutrients. Her body was too exhausted and this constant repulsion led to the inflammation at her anal passage. Traumatised at her own body's spontaneous display of such 'horrifying' symptoms and feeling helpless about NOT knowing how to end this quickly, she did not begin her school happily. Her tiny life seemed to be enveloped in fear. I still remember her desperate cry once when she murmured," Mama, I don't want this happening to me, I don't want to cry, but I can't stop it..." These unfortunate episodes continued to plague her throughout her primary school life.

In hindsight, it is interesting to note that her stress took different forms and levels over the years.

I noticed that her psychosomatic episodes would continue for at least 2 weeks into the first school term- on a daily basis! The process of going to school induced too much psychosomatic stress for her tiny body. It seemed agonising and very stressful for her to cope with the many changes that a new school term brought and this included the new environment, new teachers, new peers, new routines, new food etc. Her body could not cope with this 'self-destroying' sabotaging symptoms. While in school, her anxiety 'monster' continued to plague her – she was putting a lot of effort to control it. I found out that in her own effort of self-preservation to deal with all the stressors in school for each day in a week, she *did not* give her body a break. She did not attempt to drink any water in between classes (for she was a very timid student and didn't dare ask for permission to drink!); she did not go for toilet breaks; she did not eat during recess as it was just too stressful. She was "holding her breath" to self-preserve for the first 10 days of school! Sadly her physical body gave way to exhaustion, fatigue and anxiety. She fell very ill during her initial week in school.

During her primary school days, Tracy also struggled with her own identity. She lacked self-confidence and was as timid as a mouse in all situations. She took a really long time to warm up to her classmates and teachers. She kept all her traumas to herself and found it exceedingly difficult to verbalise her thoughts freely with any family member. Needless to say, all her fears, her bullying episodes in school and her traumatised self would surface as nightmares on most nights. She would cry and express fear of going to sleep as she was worried about waking up the next day to go school. As soon as the clock struck 11 a.m., the cycle of the psychosomatic display would become full blown!

I noticed over time, that there was a cycle of pattern about her stress manifestations. There was always a trigger for her anxiety. In her case, during that period of her life, it was everything school related and it included – meeting with teachers or friends, attending recess, the start of school terms, the start of school break terms or the period just before school started!

I observed that she would experience frequent sore throats whenever she was stressed. She would have no symptoms of a sore throat and out of the blue, a sore throat would be triggered when we were on the way to school. Another typical frequent occurrence would be her inflamed lips which looked like melted swollen goldfish lips! She would be constantly licking her chapped lips which led to an endless cycle of severely eroding of the membrane in her lip due to excessive saliva. All these symptoms are a recurrent episode of her growing anxiety. Typical triggers include social activities like the classroom show-and-tell activity, going for an interview or going for a dance performance.

In my pursuit for remedies to help her, besides the traditional psycho therapies, I searched, tested and learnt many alternative modalities to try to help her cope with that crippling anxiety condition. Honestly, I was overwhelmed with her anxiety manifestations. It was a very steep learning curve for me. I struggled to cope with her nervousness at home and in school; her lack of appetite and limited diet preferences; traumatic involuntary throwing up and the display of her irritable bowel syndrome and then incessantly wailing through numerous sleepless nights. I was at my wits end as I did not know to deal with it all. Being my first born, I was falling apart as I felt like I was not prepared at all for motherhood. My inability to tackle all these issues and at the same time balancing my career was taking a great toll on me!

I couldn't understand why these things happened and especially when the victim is a child. My heart was heavy with myriads of mixed emotions. Most of all, my whole being was swallowed in guilt as I felt that I might have passed my own stress onto her; I was angry at being 'useless' for not being able to do anything to protect her or make her suffer less. I was even questioning what the point was of having gained so much knowledge (being a psychologist helping those at work) when I could not even fix, cure or ease my own child's suffering. Internally, I was feeling great emotional pain, sorrow, frustration and even anger at my powerlessness to fix everything. I could not rest at all. This edgy feeling soon became the catalyst for my own inner search.

Along with her 'anxious energy', there were many other 'add-ons' too which appeared at different stages of her life.

As life went on, I noticed that she also exhibited an unusual level of physical attachment to valueless material items. Often, under her pillows, I would find scraps of price tags, wrappers etc that we had discarded. There'd be an emotional outburst if we ventured to remove them from her possession.

Having all comforts, we found it extremely difficult to witness her strong emotional attachment to such things of 'no-value'. Despite our objection, she would continue to keep these scraps for many moons. It did not help either when we threw them away as she would secretly pick them back!

In my search to help my daughter, I took up traditional as well as alternative self-help courses, which included Reiki, Quantum Touch, Reconnection, EFT, and Theta Healing to list a few. They were a part of my toolbox of modalities. However, by Divine timing, JSJ resonated the most to me along the way.

As Tracy's condition did not seem to improve, I decided to turn to JSJ as a last resort. Being a new student of this art, my knowledge of applying the variety of steps or flows overwhelmed me. I felt I was not proficient enough in doing all the complicated flows. However, I was determined to commit to doing the flows regularly. All I cared and wanted was for Tracy to be well and harmonised. I really wanted to put an end to those horrible feelings she was experiencing as a stressed-out being. Upon commitment, for the next 21 days, during the period of the year-end school holidays, I would tip toe into her room while she was sleeping. Using only a small torch light and referring to the JSJ texts, I would follow the steps in the text and commit one hour daily session during the early morning hours, afternoon and night. I did not know what to expect but I knew I had to do something. I was holding the fingers-and-toes flow and first depth flows.

Using the self-help steps daily, she slowly began to sleep better, eat better and she seemed to feel more at ease. Her chronic psychosomatic symptoms of frequent nightmares, daily involuntary vomiting and irritable bowel syndrome just before the school bus arrived gradually dissipated. That irritating attachment and need to collect scraps disappeared over time. Her mental state is now no longer like some would say, 'kan-cheong' or a nervous mess of emotions. She now seems to be able to discard what is not serving her well at the mind, body and spirit level. Her frequent stressed related episodes of sore throats have drastically reduced. She is able to handle the 'unknown' or uncertainty of situations more calmly without any of those psychosomatic symptoms. With the release of all that was negative stress, her heart has now seemed to have created space for love and affection. She is much more responsive and able to verbalise details during conversations. She begun to give hugs and be allowed to be hugged. Although it was not instant, these incremental improvements were noticeable over time. Tracy is much more at ease with herself now and within her own skin. After rigorous JSJ hands flow, she has finally been able to focus on her journey in life now.

It was a slow transformation but, she has grown from being a timid little mousy girl to a confident, intuitive and kind teen.

In support of how JSJ transformed her, it is only correct if I list some of her own accomplishments:

- The progress she has made as a ballet dancer is amazing.
- She achieved a junior black belt in taekwondo .... Within two years, she had 2 double promotions in her grading and reached the black belt title by age 11, and competed and won national competitions.

Fast forward to the present moment, Tracy is a happy and spirit free being now. She possesses an aura of serenity and calmness, and this is such a stark contrast to the past.

The journey with my daughter has transformed me too. I had to learn how to undo most of the preconceived knowledge that I had. I learnt to let go of the need to ensure myself that things were happening the way I or society felt was the 'right' way. I had to trust in the process and in doing so, I learnt to deal with my own anxiety and to let go of the need to control how I would like the outcome to be. For that, I am very thankful.

Way to go Tracy! Mama's wish for you is to Grow with life and enjoy your journey ahead!

A Note to Myself:

I have learnt to become a fierce advocate of healing through touch since I became a first time mom. It is essential to have Patience, Belief and Trust. Tracy and I are now transformed to a great extent and the process has been beneficial to us.

Being in this competitive societal culture, I have witnessed numerous stressful childhood traumas amongst our Singaporean kids. The pressure of Singaporean parenthood in trying to ensure our kids are among the 'top' cohort or at least not falling behind others and the need to keep up with the 'so-called' competency lists for our kids from as young as in preschool. It is this awareness that my hubby and I are always mindful in ensuring that our kids DO NOT get caught in this rat race. We value their harmony and 'sanity over pseudo-superiority". We recognise that there is really no point in 'forcing' or packing our child's life's schedules with myriads of activities when the individual is holistically not ready. When the body (physical, mental-emotional) is not ready, we need to exercise care and discretion to decide what are the TRUE higher -order priorities to take place first.

I am confident that whatever stress her little body might have experienced since the in-uteral period (and or due to my pregnancy stress), each layer of stress which may be locked into her tissue memory, has been removed, released and her body is now harmonised.

I also learned that True healing is transformative and lasting. Healing takes time and commitment. I learnt that I should not dictate or expect the way I want the healing outcome to be. In doing so, I may have (often!) missed out on what was going on then. There were many times when I felt that NOTHING BIG was happening after many countless weeks of sessions. In fact, nothing was happening and I could not see with my physical eyes what I was hoping to see. During those moments of utter despair and frustration, I could not appreciate the 'nothingness' that took place for many weeks, and even months. I remembered how one time, I was actually frustrated and angry that the fever my child was having (at 38.9 degrees!) did not subside even after medication and our JSJ session.

In retrospect, it DID make a great difference to her! Even though she was still having a high fever, after the JSJ session, she was no longer lying motionless and in great discomfort (which she would normally be). She was running around playing with our dog! JSJ did help her *adapt* to her own situation!

As time progressed, I saw that the changes were very subtle but sure. The changes that take place are for real and the change is constantly evolving.

I am truly thankful to have embraced JSJ as it has helped my daughter tremendously in her journey. From my first-hand experience with my daughter, I then embarked on my own journey with JSJ!

Case 2 – My 'Ah-Ha' moment with JSJ

As I was attached to a special school early in my career, the opportunity to utilize JSJ was presented to me one day in 2009. Mary, a 12-yr old was diagnosed with ADHD and has a history of rebellious behaviours. She was admitted to the special school since young. Coming from a disadvantaged background, Mary had never seen or experienced her parents' love and care. They had left her at a very young age and she was cared for by her aging grandmother who could not manage her disruptive behaviour.

Mary had good social communication skills and responded well to praises and encouragement. However, there was one particular year, when she was often sent out of class for counselling with one of my colleagues. I noticed and sensed that there seemed to have been a mismatch in the profiles between the class form teacher with Mary and many other students. I had even forewarned the management team about this scenario before the allocation and placement of teachers for the following year. Unfortunately no one listened and took me seriously.

In fact, there was an increase in 'mischief and misbehaviour' in that particular class where Mary was placed in. Her behavioural outbursts became more frequent and severe and almost every day she was sent to the counselling room! I hated to see that the good foundation which all the therapists had laid over the years seemed to be destroyed by this 'mismatch' overnight. It pained me to see this poor child struggling to stay afloat with such a challenging form teacher. Not heeding professional advice is a situation many of us could have faced at times.

In that same year, Mary was also prescribed Ritalin, by the psychiatrist to help her manage her sudden increase outbursts in school. My colleague was tasked with the assignment of administering this drug to her during recess. At the pantry where we sometimes met over a cup of tea, I would often tease him that he was like a 'puppet' dispensing a 'magic' potion which would drastically alter things for the better. He would add the medication into a cup of Milo and give it to her. So the 'job' was completed!

I would remind him about the dangers of overdosing the child without proper monitoring and the effectiveness of the dosage. The relevant personnel had to monitor such prescriptions carefully to see its effectiveness.

One hot afternoon, while all the paramedical therapists were out for lunch, Mary stormed into the office and desperately shouted out aloud, "Please help me!" There was no one else in the office except me, and I knew I had to help her. I quickly laid her down on a bed at the sick bay, removed her shoes, and I started our JSJ session. I did a fingers-and-toes flow. (Again this flow! Because there is the only flow I could do without referring to the texts at that time of my learning journey!:)

At that moment, when I placed my hands on her, I felt that her body was as cold as ice and as tense as bowstring. It seemed like thick steel armour had wrapped tightly all around her body. Her true self seemed to be encased in a hard shell. Her face was beetroot red and big droplets of perspiration dotted her forehead. Her blouse seemed drenched. Her fists were clenched, and she seemed ready to administer a punch at anyone who was in her way.

Minutes into the session, she was also exclaiming that there were spiders crawling all over her back and hands. She was cringing on her back like an overturned dried leaf and shaking her hands forcefully every few minutes to shake the spiders off her hands. I guessed that it was probably the long term side-effects of the medication.

During the initial 10 minutes, she would continue to cringe and curl her body up and cry over spiders on her back. I continued to distract her by engaging her in a conversation about food and her love for cooking. 'Magically', within 20 minutes, in the midst of the JSJ session, she became more relaxed and we could focus more on the conversation till the end of the session. Her terrible anxiety and tension seemed to have 'melted' away. *It was such a powerful yet humbling moment for me to experience and witness how JSJ brings harmony (physical, mental, spiritual) to our body.*

"Cher, you did magic!", she said as she left smiling in a calmed and composed state. She was almost like a different person in a different 'state'.

By the time the whole episode was over, my colleagues who had returned from their lunch breaks exclaimed in disbelief that I had successfully spent an hour with her. To this, that moment spent with Mary, sends shivers down my spine...reminding me of the importance of being able to rebalance and harmonize ourselves when our body is 'out-of-balance' in mind, body or spirit.

A Note to myself:

Our Body is an amazing machine! Healing IS possible at all levels. JSJ harmonises our inner sync and brings about the desired balance meant for our body at that moment in time. Unlike traditional medications, which stimulates or sedates, JSJ allows internal adjustment to happen entirely on its own. We just have to be the willing 'hands'.

(*My personal view on prescribing medication on students is that although I understand the great benefits of medication, personally, I do NOT support prescribing medication on anyone especially young students without having the proper and detailed process to monitor or review the cases individually. I have seen many unfortunate cases while I was working as a psychologist in schools. NOT only do they NOT get weaned off the medications prescribed, they have to live with many horrible side effects which no one can help rectify. Relying on medication alone IS NOT the only heavenly way out.)

Case 3 – My Papa my humbling moment with JSJ

My beloved Papa was 83 years old when he was diagnosed with terminal cancer. Between 2013-2014, he was admitted several times into hospital for complications relating to his respiratory organs, liver and spleen. He spent 5 months in the intensive care unit. In addition to all the complications, he had a painful tracheostomy which involved a surgical procedure on the anterior part of his neck. The doctors had to insert a tube into his windpipe to help him breathe better.

My world literally came to a halt with that. My waking and sleeping moments were filled with thoughts of him and no one else. Even my own family – my husband and my two girls took a back seat in my life. I told my two girls that their loving 'Ah Kong' was to be my baby, as he needed my attention, care and time. I am still very grateful and thankful that my girls would join me in holding the flows together whenever we visited him then.

When I reflect back on the situation, I felt that my mental focus then was as if I was preparing for a battle. Throughout that period, I did not allow my emotions to drown out my momentum to help him heal. I didn't stop to entertain or allow my emotions to drag me down. I was 'numb' to some extent and didn't have time to entertain intense emotions. I executed the control of my emotions so expertly, that I didn't even cry at his funeral! Before the illness took him away, I was preserving my sanity for what was needed for him. Like engaging in warfare, I picked out controlled emotions that were necessary to tackle what was needed. I needed to conserve myself to keep going and attend to him as long as and as often as it was needed. I didn't have the time or the energy to assist my family with anything. I felt like I was the solitary soldier battling an unknown enemy!

Every day, I would spend my time thinking of what flows to do for him and I studied the pages of notes I had scribbled during the classes I attended over the years. I wanted him to live... I was not ready to let him go! I used all the knowledge I had acquired and the materials I had gained from JSJ to help and support his journey. Using my hands daily on simple JSJ sequences, I was able to relieve the pain and any discomfort he felt.

Despite all the medical attention he received in the hospital, there were numerous "emergency" encounters, but JSJ brought great release to him at those moments of despair and helplessness. During one of my hospital visits when Papa was in the ICU, I noticed that the blood pressure monitor showed a reading of 200+. There was no one to attend to him immediately and so while waiting for help, I remembered a flow which I had learnt to lower high blood pressure readings. I quickly started holding Papa's arm and at the same time kept a close watch on the readings on the monitor. I was also praying in my heart for the Divine to work through me to bring the highest harmony for him. When I finally finished the last step of the flow, lo and behold, the BP reading was brought down to 120!

There was yet another incident where the timely intervention of JSJ helped. It was during one of my routine visits in the early afternoon. I was surprised to see the hospital's "lung specialist" attending to my Papa. The specialist was forcefully "squeezing" Papa's chest several times and watching a monitor. He repeated these actions several times. I walked up to him and asked him what was happening. The specialist replied that Papa's oxygen reading on the monitor was low and that he needed attention. I figured out that he was trying to induce better respiratory intake but the monitor screen was still showing no sign of any change or improvement in his oxygen level. It stayed at only 68%.

As I watched the specialist continue his 'squeezing' protocol, I wanted to help my Papa too. I walked over to the end of the bed and gently placed my fingers on his toes. I remembered with JSJ, that one of the toes helps with breath. I thought that such a simple act would not cause any harm. I had no expectation when holding his toes but to only send love and harmony... that was my only intention for Papa. I remembered holding onto both his middle toes.

Miraculously, the oxygen reading on the monitor started to increase steadily! It went from 68% to 75% and then steadily reached 99%. My heart was pounding non-stopped and I was feeling elated with this outcome! I continued to monitor his reading throughout the whole day.

The 99% reading remained throughout the day. Another day with my Papa that I was so grateful for.

As my Papa's stay in the hospital extended for many weeks, and he lay inert, there were days when he could not clear his bowels. He would express his great discomfort to me when I visited him. The prescribed medication didn't help either and he felt his digestive tract greatly congested. He was badly constipated. As he lay on the bed, I placed my hands on his calves and 'palmed' them for about 10-15 minutes as a step to help with constipation. I noticed that the visitors at a nearby bed slowly began moving out of the room. He was letting off smelly flatulence and could finally "let go" after many days of severe constipation! That was indeed a release and relief!

Towards the latter end of his journey, Papa expressed his wish to be home for the Lunar New Year and he did not want to be in hospice care either. With great effort, we finally brought him home to continue with his palliative care. The hospice staff visited us and suggested the possible use of morphine if he needed it as a last resort to manage his condition. We did not use any throughout his journey.

We transformed his bedroom into a "mini-ICU" with a hospital bed, portable and adjustable commode, ventilator and drips stand etc. I even got for him an ice-cream bell to alert us if he needed attention!

Once home, Papa didn't have the hospital's round-the-clock care he had there. Hence, we, as a family including the helper, became the 24/7 care team. It was very trying and exhausting for all of us. To be honest, I did not have time to let any emotions take up any space in my mind and heart. I was in a race against time and time was of the essence. I had to be the daily 'jump start cable' for him to help him cope with his situation. My waking and sleeping moments were just thoughts about what I could do to make him feel better and live better every minute.

Some of the challenging conditions as a caregiver included flipping and changing Papa's lying position often so that he did not get any sores. My Papa was a big built man who was at least 1.8 m tall and weighing over 90 kg. Another necessary task was periodically sticking the sucking apparatus into his throat to suck out any mucus, fluid or secretions blocking his airways. The airways had to be always clear for easy breathing. This was the one task that I could not personally administer. Our helpers were good and I have to thank them for being ever so patient, caring and watchful over papa's needs.

Some weeks after being home, I observed that Papa had suddenly lost his voice and his hearing too. But this was probably due to his tracheostomy. Papa was still mentally alert and he would hand signal his discomfort and I would try to communicate with him through drawing, writing and speaking. For the next 2 weeks I started doing flows intensively. I recalled what the instructor had shared about JSJ and being able to reverse a disharmony. If applied as early as the onset, it can harmonise and remove the problem totally. I just wanted to help Papa feel a little better each day.

With this hope in my heart, I faithfully gave him JSJ sessions for the next 14 days. During one of the sessions, Papa was waving his hands at me signalling that his throat area was in pain while I was doing the flows. I assured Papa that it was a good sign that the energy was moving and healing in that area. The following week, Papa surprised me by calling my mobile and chatted briefly with me. That moment I heard his voice, it brought tears of gratefulness to my eyes. I thanked the Divine profusely!

As we prepared for the onset of the Lunar New Year 2014 at home, Papa was also trying to wean off the reliance on the ventilator. Given his tracheostomy, his breathing had to be supported by a mechanical ventilator 24/7. Hence we rented one. Papa had to be attached to this 'life-breather' at all times. The ventilator was supposed to suck and filter out the oxygen from his surroundings and pump it back into his lung through the tracheostomy tube. There were times when the signals at the ventilator kept beeping due to some errors and we had to scramble for help to troubleshoot! We managed to get past those technical hiccups with the help and support from family, friends and the support team from hospital.

With the doctor's recommendation, we tried to wean him off his reliance on the ventilator. We helped Papa carry out his breathing exercises, and we continued our daily JSJ sessions. The focus now was on helping to strengthen his respiratory system. It was a gradual improvement. At the start, Papa could wean off the ventilator for only 5 mins and then gradually to 10 and 20 minutes daily before being reattached to the ventilator. Surely but slowly, we noticed that he could stand alone and breathe without the ventilator for up to an hour a day for the initial week. Subsequently he did it for up to three hours a day! Another miracle to be grateful for!

Despite all these improvements, Papa left us peacefully on the morning of 9 June 2014. Throughout his journey, he did not rely on the morphine which was given as an alternative by the hospice nurse. Thanks to JSJ, he did not suffer any pain. In fact, that beautiful morning, just before he left us, there was a ray of transient light that hovered around his feet. This beautiful calming light then moved over to his crown and brought Papa's spirit up... Papa was smiling on his bed. I really do not know the significance of this but I am sure Papa is now with the Light!

It was indeed a humbling experience to see how JSJ had helped in the major moments of pain and discomfort; and how it brought small moments of peace and relief that led to big moments of family connection with him. I still miss him dearly but looking back, I am glad to have been there for him, and I'm thankful that I had a companion in JSJ to keep me positive unconditionally. In my humble opinion, not only did JSJ extend his lifespan and relieved his pain (he didn't need to resort to any morphine to manage his discomfort), it also supported him in the process of dying, with little struggle and pain. To me, JSJ transformed what could have been a lonely journey into a dignified experience for my Papa. Just like JSJ, he was returned to harmony and that itself is JSJ. Thank you from the bottom of my heart JSJ!

Case 4 – Pebbles, my miniature Schnauzer

Pebbles, my 15-year-old schnauzer, passed away in 2015. She was a courageous beauty who fought the good fight to the end. Pebbles was diagnosed with illnesses linked with old age and she was hospitalised for weeks due to innumerable complications.

Towards the end of her life, her kidneys were failing and she had severe skin problems. The eczema often led to unhealed, painful and raw wounds which 'grew' up to the size of a palm. It was agonizing to see patches of skin, sore with redness dropping off at times from her body! The wounds remained raw and wet for many weeks as it could not heal with the medication the vet had prescribed. I could not brush, pat or even stroke her for fear that my lightest and softest touch would cause another patch to drop off.

Sadly condition did not get better even with intense professional medical help and a week of hospitalisation. Instinctively, I decided to apply JSJ on her raw wounds. I placed my right palm just above the wounded area and my left palm onto my right hand for at least 20 minutes daily. To my surprise, it started to heal. New skin grew after one week! Pebbles left peacefully with all her wounds healed and a new layer of skin. Thank you JSJ for restoring her body before she crossed over!

Case 5 – My adventure with an injured pigeon

During one of my nature walks, I stumbled upon an injured pigeon. It lay motionless on the ground with its head tucked unnaturally near its feet. Stooping down to have a closer look, I noted that the poor pigeon seemed to have fallen off a tree and although still alive it was barely moving as it could not 'undo' its contorted body. I was in a dilemma for a while, as I wasn't sure if I could take the pigeon home to care for it as I had never nursed a bird back to health! However, I decided very quickly to do so, when I saw a maid with two ferocious looking dogs heading in the same way. I did not wish for the pigeon to be in their way. Hurriedly, I picked it up with a plastic bag I found nearby and took it home.

I examined it carefully as I cleaned it with a solution made from sea salt. There was blood on its tongue and left eyelid which I gently wiped. It's left eye seemed to be bulging out of its socket! There was also some injury to its wings. The pigeon seemed to be in bad shape. Without hesitation, I applied JSJ onto the pigeon for 20 minutes and it did not move or struggle at all. After that, it miraculously began to move its head, body and wings instantaneously and started to walk a few steps! Encouraged by this speedy recovery, I applied JSJ again after a few hours. By then, it flapped its wings and was hopping about in the small basket I had prepared.

After the second JSJ session, the pigeon flew around my house and landed onto the balcony window. I knew it was well and time for it to go. Before it flew off, the pigeon instinctively looked back at my family as if saying thank you and acknowledging the help for a good 20 seconds. We bade it goodbye as it seemed to take a deep breath, spread its wings and flew to the tall swaying trees outside our balcony. I was grateful for the opportunity to assist this creature. Although small, it enriched my experience.

Case 6 – First mental-emotional case, restored

In 2009, when I was working as a psychologist and practising JSJ as a free-lance basis, I encountered Kee Kee who was my first mental-emotional case. Kee Kee, a professional in her mid-thirties, moved to Singapore from China.

She shared that over a span of 5 years, she had moved more than seven times across different countries due to her husband's career. They had two young children and both of preschool age. She had a successful career as an accountant but decided to quit her job to care for her family and especially for one of her kids who was diagnosed with autism. Due to their constant moves across countries, she faced very limited support from friends and family who were stationed in her home country.

Her husband was holding a high post in MNC and would often come home late due to his work commitments. As a result of that, there was constant strain on their marital relationship. Not being able to take the strain of being a sole caregiver, she was diagnosed with depression and displayed suicidal tendencies. She was prescribed medication by a psychiatrist and had to work with an in-house psychologist. As she was not very satisfied with only consuming medication, Kee Kee sought out JSJ as an additional support therapy.

While each session of JSJ brought different kinds of relief and healing for Kee Kee, there were moments where she experienced a lot of pain and numbness in her limbs and body. I remembered on one occasion, Kee Kee reported that there were bruises that mysteriously surfaced on the upper side of her face after the session. When probed further about her past, she revealed that when she was in her teens, she was sexually abused by a relative. She recalled an encounter that was violent where her head was held tightly and banged against the wall. I observed that these past unhealed wounds and trauma are being 'dispersed' or 'dissolved' as seen in the mysterious bruises being surfaced up and clearing over the next few days.

Despite the fact that her progress to her healing seemed slow, she would faithfully turn up for the sessions. She was determined to help herself heal. One consistent observation was, after each session, Kee

Kee would come out more cheerful, positive and aware of her situation. She seems to have a better awareness cognitively despite the sedative medication and was able to surmount strength to move on with her life despite all the marital struggles she was facing. After about a few months, Kee Kee told me she had found a job as a preschool teacher. She has moved on with her life.

With Kee Kee, I learnt that JSJ has the power to heal old wounds and injuries – at the mind, body and spirit level. Healing becomes the priority when JSJ is administered. It clears and heals old wounds before the healing goes up to the next level. Not all healing is visible. Medications for such conditions like anxiety or depression, sedates or stimulates. However, JSJ seeks to harmonise and regulate the circulation within the body; it brings the body up to the appropriate level of harmonising at that moment in time.

Case 7 – A disharmony reversed to a harmonious state

Amongst all my cases to date, Joey was one of the most challenging yet mind blowing experiences for me. In 2015, I responded to a mother's whatsapp message to help her daughter. My heart was drawn to her whatsapp profile message which read … "I need a miracle".

Joey was about 8 years old when we started our JSJ journey together. She is a special needs child with a history of severe epilepsy. Fortunately for her, she has a very loving and supportive family where her parents, younger brother and grandparents tirelessly care for her needs.

Her young brother who is five, is a great gift from the Divine. Despite his tender age and small size, he has a beautiful aura of great maturity around him. He is the sweetest and most adorable boy I have encountered. While most five years old kids would be playing and seeking attention for his own needs and wants, he spends his time attending to his older sister's needs and he helps his mother with the household chores too. He has learnt to accommodate and constantly gives in to his Jie Jie (big sister) who he understands to be a special needs child, and plays an active supporting role to the family.

Epilepsy Floods

From the age of three, and after many episodes of having a high fever, Joey's childhood life started to fall apart. For over eight years, the web of epilepsy entangled her deeply as each day passed. She had about 100 episodic attacks DAILY! (Yes, it is Not a typo error nor an exaggeration!). As a result of this frequency, her cognitive functioning as well as her developmental progress were severely impacted. Her mother's life to date is unequally devoted to her and most of her time revolves around caring for Joey. In desperation, the family sought numerous ways – traditional and non-traditional healings including various modalities hoping to find some relief for her.

With the traditional medical intervention method, they had tried most of the anti-epileptic drugs. She was also on a ketogenic diet as recommended by one of her doctors. However, this treatment was abandoned weeks after they found such approach very detrimental to her kidneys and she was reduced to bones. Joey was also advised to take a dosage of 30 tablets of pyridoxal 5' phosphate (P-5-P) daily. This treatment was very challenging to her care-giver, as many hours were spent 'forcing' the tablets into her or 'enticing' her to swallow them all, one by one. Despite all this, her body did not respond well to the recommended treatments from the medical front. The family then decided to stop all medical intervention treatments. The medical specialist had condescendingly remarked that Joey might never get off the epilepsy attacks completely if they choose to stop the treatment. They were in greater despair.

Joey had also attended whole brain learning therapy, speech and occupational therapy. The family had even sought spiritual help as they were desperate. The frequency and episodes of the epilepsy attacks she had each day seemed more challenging than the last. Her sleep pattern was always erratic, she would sleep very late in the night and wake up after a few hours of sleep and that too at the wee hours of the morning. Her temperament was extremely unpredictable and uncontrollable. Having to feed her 30 tablets daily was another challenge that was exhaustive. Going out for a simple social event was almost impossible for her family or at least for her fatigued mother. Her mother shared that she had become so used to or accustomed to the cruel stares or even judgemental scorns by the strangers who did not understand Joey especially when she was in a meltdown situation. She has learnt to remain calm in spite of all. As a very hot headed person, Joey's mother shared that caring for Joey had drastically changed her life. Joey has taught her to be extremely patient and 'thick-skinned' too in the face of a judging crowd.

Unfortunately for Joey, as her unpredictable and erratic sleeping behaviour worsened, none of her family members could have a peaceful night's rest. All these challenges made it difficult for her to continue in the special school she was attending. She was unfortunately 'phased out' of that special school. This meant that Joey was now at home 24/7 and nobody could actually get a good rest! That was yet another additional burden on the care-giver. According to Joey's mother, those periods were her "darkest and lowest moment..."

JSJ treatments

Joey started JSJ in 2015 and both her family and I had barely any expectations. Our JSJ sessions over the next twenty months or so were like tug-of-war sessions! It was a struggle between the adults and her. A typical session would be Joey screaming, yelling and shouting at the top of her voice and kicking me out of the sofa on which we were working on. On better days, she would be sleeping in her bunk bed and kicking me occasionally when she awoke. Our JSJ sessions happened anywhere that she would lay on for that day. I would sit on the narrow edge of the double decker stairs attached to the bed, on the sofa or on the floor. Often, she would shout in her sleep or throw a flying kick from the bunk bed during the session. Many would consider such behaviour as intolerable, however, I chose to put on a different lens. To me, she was a child struggling with inner disharmony and crying out for help. I prayed the most whenever I had sessions with her. Oftentimes, I would seek Divine and ask if I should continue this therapy for her. Deep down I wanted to continue the therapy as I knew that Healing can be invisible.

Joey's mother and I developed an understanding over time that we were on this journey to support her recovery. She would even trust me to be alone with Joey while she took a short respite, by doing her grocery shopping or marketing. Over the years, Joey's mother has developed this cool and calm disposition to handle all of Joey's 'commotions' that she has faced daily. For a number of months, our JSJ sessions were always conducted in an enclosed room with all windows closed for fear that her outbursts would disturb the whole neighbourhood.

The progress Joey made initially was very subtle and I continued to encourage her mother to see the little differences and changes Joey was making. Even when we noted that the frequency of her epilepsy attacks had reduced, Joey's mom was exceedingly apprehensive to acknowledge that – for FEAR that it might jinx it all. So to ease the tension, we would 'tip toe' around that topic and not openly talk about it.. This was because the family had been disappointed on numerous occasions over the years and Joey's mother chose to keep silent or pretend the situation was unchanging, that is, 'pretend indifference with fingers crossed silently in her heart'. It was a way to maintain self-preservation.

After about 2 years, we noticed that her temperament had improved tremendously! Her screaming and aggressive outbursts were gradually replaced with a calm and positive state of being. She seemed to have transcended out of that 'mental' state which often deluded me where one moment she would be screaming and at the very next instant she would be laughing and talking to herself or with an invisible being. Joey's mother and I chose to recognise that when such moments occurred, we assumed that Joey was having a conversation with the Higher Divine. To date, her state of being is definitely more 'present' and loving towards her family members. She has over time developed more comprehensive speech and can carry out a good conversation for a prolonged period of time! Her vocabulary range has also increased and suddenly we are now greeted with rich vocabulary which her mind had absorbed since birth. Another joyful improvement I have witnessed is that Joey enjoys playing and engaging in purposeful tasks such as looking for books to read and write, and even working on puzzles. What a beautiful outcome! Most wonderful of all is that her episodic attacks have ended COMPLETELY despite her medical specialist still being sceptical of her recovery! Both Joey's mother and I would like to recognise that all the little 'miracles' have been made possible with the help of all the therapies she had gone through. After three years of JSJ therapy, I am very grateful to be part of Joey's journey. She is still making great progress and is attending another special school.

A recent message which Joey's mother shared is that she is doing well and helping her granny with house chores. She has grown much taller and has managed to put on weight successfully now! Her mother too has gone back to work.

I wish her all the BEST in her many happy new milestones to come. Indeed JOY to the world!

What I have learnt
Joey's mother, Anna, over the years displayed an unassailable spirit. Her unbreakable fortitude gave me strength too. I have to thank her for

showing me the power and strength of a mother's love. Despite all the setbacks she faced, she devoted and sacrificed her time, effort and love over all the years to care for her loved ones. Despite the constant lack of sleep and great fatigue she felt, she still had the strength to care for both her children. She has raised her son Joe, in the best way she could. She taught him to care for others, especially his big Jie Jie (sister), to give in to her demands willingly and happily even at such a young age. She has indeed raised such a pair of lovely kids!

I have also learnt that whatever stage of disharmony the body is facing, there is always something good JSJ can offer to do.

Like the changing of the seasons of nature – there is a time for 'release/remove', 'repair' and 'regenerate'. I have learnt that when the body is READY – it will take in nutrients, digest and utilise it appropriately. There is no point in flushing or flooding the body (mind, body and spirit) with more than what it can handle.

JSJ works to cleanse when it is necessary and in this case I feel it sees that as the foremost priority before it can build and boost. It is interesting to note that with the improvement in her mental state and temperaments, there were also some significant physical changes we observed. One obvious improvement is the hard protrusion on her inner arcs in her feet, which she developed since birth, had disappeared completely. It is no longer visible along her arc. In JSJ, this area corresponds to the Safety Energy Lock No. 6 (SEL 6), which anchors and holds our structure firm and erect. It is a symbol of Balance.

Thank you JSJ, for bringing balance and harmony to her mental-emotional state. Thinking back, I felt the power of this message.

From over hundred counts of daily epilepsy attacks to ZERO... indeed a MIRACLE has occurred!

Case 8 – Let there be light!

Uncle Sean, aged 70, was admitted to a hospital due to retinal detachment on his left eye. Although the operation went smoothly, it did not guarantee full vision recovery. According to the doctors at the hospital, a percentage of patients sadly were at high risk of losing their vision despite the operation.

It was a painful post-op recovery journey for him. As per medical advice and the follow up, he had to maintain a 'face down' position **at all times** to prevent putting extra pressure on his eye. He was also warned against lifting any heavy objects or doing any strenuous activity. During his waking and sleeping moments, his posture was a challenge to manage, it was equally agonising to keep his head facing down but it was necessary to maintain that posture to avoid any other complications. This whole event before and after the operation, brought about a great deal of stress and it slowly developed into fear for him and his family. He had to remain warded at the hospital although he wanted very much to go home to recuperate.

Due to the slow progress of healing, a new complication arose, Uncle Sean could not be discharged from hospital. He had developed the inability to urinate and was in distress. The recommendation was to insert a catheter to closely monitor his situation. The very thought of having a catheter inserted into him created more stress! Every few hours, a bladder scan was carried out and with each scan, Uncle Sean was greeted with great disappointment. He was also in great pain and he wanted out!

As the family was desperate to get him discharged, they decided to try JSJ. Interestingly, within two short periods of time of JSJ treatment, Uncle Sean was getting up more often than before to urinate! Shortly after, while still holding the JSJ poses, he started wetting the bed before he could make his way to the bathroom in time. That was a BIG 'relief' for him – to his bladder and his emotions too! He was discharged the same day, as he showed improvement and his family and I were amazed at how quickly we witnessed the results! It was truly an eye opener for Uncle Sean who is usually sceptical about unconventional therapy.

A month later, Uncle Sean was due for his first post operative eye check-up. They waited with bated breath hoping he could at least regain some vision. When the doctor shared the outcome, all their hearts sank. He could not see anything at all despite the surgery to reattach his retina. The family sought my advice and guidance. Both the family and Uncle Sean were diligent in doing the 'homework' I gave them on a daily basis.

A few weeks later, Uncle Sean went for his second follow up appointment for his eye. Everyone was gloating with happiness as his eye condition had improved in leaps and bounds! His vision was even better than before his operation! Uncle Sean is now a true believer of JSJ and he does the self help poses himself daily for his overall well-being.

Case 9 – Let's sing a song!

Zack was one of earliest cases with Down Syndrome. He was a preschooler with very limited speech. His family members were very supportive of his developmental needs and they were positive about JSJ therapy. They were hoping for Zack to be admitted into a mainstream school and be able to remain in that environment coping well. As a psychologist with the Ministry of Education and special school, I had witnessed numerous cases of special needs children being streamed out of mainstream schools at a young age. Very few similar cases do eventually make it through the mainstream schools system, with LOTS of support from ALL involved.

During our initial weekly sessions, Zack was usually quiet and did not interact very much. He was very obedient and would happily lay down on the therapy bed throughout the sessions. After a few sessions, while I was singing the nursery rhymes during the session, he opened his mouth and started singing the nursery rhymes with me! We were very encouraged and delighted with this outburst! As we saw progress, his parents were encouraged by the outcome and they continued diligently with the 'homework' as Zack continued his weekly JSJ session.

The following year, Zack started his primary school journey in a mainstream school and he coped well!

With JSJ, Zack continues to sing his own songs and progresses well!

Case 10 – Supple muscles for Baby R

Baby R was my youngest case. He was 18 months old when we started JSJ therapy. On the day of Baby R's birth, his twin brother sadly passed on. Baby R was born with profound hearing loss and diagnosed as having dystonia cerebral palsy. Being born a premature baby at 27 weeks, he barely weighed 850 grams. Before the age of one, he had already undergone and braved five operations.

Baby R had extremely tense muscle tone over all of his body which required steroid and muscle relaxant medication. The muscles on the left side of his body from his face to his toes are very rigid and tensed. Being 'pigeon-chested', his sternum still protrudes forward and outward causing an uneven tension on his chest wall. Thus, he tended to have difficulty breathing and often breathed through his mouth. He had great difficulty bending or flexing his elbow to control his movements, such as putting a pacifier into his mouth. We also noticed that his head was pulled to the left and he was unable to turn his head to his right side. He was also presented with poor or reduced oculomotor control on his left eye and this atypical eye was significantly noticeable. Despite all these, Baby R was a gentle fighter with great spirit.

I saw Baby R twice weekly for therapy and I gave his family 'homework' to do as a follow up. About two weeks later, we noted interesting progress. We noticed that his overall muscles seemed to have loosened up and he could turn his neck to both sides without having to turn his whole body when he wanted to look at the therapist!

After another week of JSJ treatment, Baby R continued to make slow but good progress! Given his cerebral palsy condition at the beginning, his family became worried that his tensed up muscles would become a problem for him again. However to our relief, his muscular tone continued to remain supple and soft! He could raise both of his arms and elbows. He was able to raise and flex his arms with better control and relaxation. The tension on his neck started to gradually ease when he lay on his bed. He could turn to look at people from both sides too! After some time, he was off steroids as well as the relaxant medication for his muscles. Interestingly, we also noticed that his left eye was becoming more 'normal'. Visually, he was making better eye tracking and it became less obvious as a deficiency. Such a significant observation was also noted by the medical team.

Baby R is now 4 years old. We started JSJ sessions in 2017 from the beginning of his fragile life. He has made tremendous progress. In spite of many challenges, Baby R's parents remain very loving and patient in their care for Baby R. Baby R may still have a long road towards recovery, but JSJ has contributed immensely in his initial fragility phase of life. Keep going Baby R!

Case 11 – Breakthrough after decades

I met Yanni, a professional, when she was in her thirties. Her involvement in setting up the private firm she worked for was pivotal since its conception. To date, she has been one of the most competent and diligent professionals I had ever met. She devoted her time tirelessly to her work and she put in long weary hours without complaints. For over 15 years, she remained a faithful and devoted worker at that company she helped kick start.

Despite many years of rigorous and conscientious hard work, her unflagging effort was not well appreciated. She was weighed down immensely by emotional blackmail by her boss and this included verbal abuse too. Her family and close friends had advised her (but without success) over the decades that it was time for her to leave the workplace. They were at their wits end because they had 'put up' with her eon years of procrastination. Deep inside her heart, Yanni knew that was the best option for her but she just could not find the courage to leave. Each time she tried to tender her resignation, she found herself trapped in an endless emotionally 'blackmailed' maze. She had retracted her resignation many times. When she wanted to walk away, she just could not gather enough courage to do it. She kept postponing the chapter for happiness in her life to later date. She kept prioritising her workplace responsibilities before hers. Her melancholic state continued to affect her deeply as she had to bear and absorb the abuses.

In time, she began struggling with numbness and pain on her left thigh. She was in great discomfort, and could no longer sit for long stretches. She had to constantly shift her body weight every few minutes to cope with the pain. This tremendously affected her focus and ability to work. Coincidentally, besides her physical dis-ease; at work, she felt like she was 'frozen' in her career path. Thus, she was being weighed down with a tidal wave of frustrations.

To tackle the pain and numbness in her lower part of her body, Yanni went for electro-therapy as was recommended by a friend. It relieved the pain but only temporarily. Soon the numbness and pain returned. At this point of her life, she felt like her condition was beyond therapy as the level of numbness was too excruciating for her to bear.

After much contemplation, Yanni decided to try JSJ as what felt like a last resort. Being her first timer, she described it as a "mind-blowing experience!" after the first session.

Yanni was very alert and conversant during all the sessions. With a super sensitive body that could sense and trace the flow or pathway of the energy within her, she shared that she felt a lot of energy moving within her body. During the initial sessions, an interesting observation would take place. Within minutes in the sessions, her body would start to relax and she would feel a surge of the energy in both her thighs. On naked eyes, it looked like both her thighs would involuntarily vibrate vigorously. This process reminded me of the technique called Tremor/Tension Release Exercise created by Dr David Berceli, an expert in trauma intervention.

It seems that Yanni's cumulative repression of her physical, emotional and mental stress/trauma, which often is stored in tissue memory, was being released through tremors and shaking. It has been well researched that shaking is a primal impulse to a stressful situation and it is our natural body response to bringing back to normal homeostasis.

Almost immediately after the first session ended, she was eager to test the effectiveness of this therapy. She jumped off the bed instantly, moving and lifting her legs up without any difficulty. To her surprise (and mine too!), the pain along her lower back and thighs were completely gone! Interestingly after the session, and over the weekend, Yanni burped non-stop! She felt a lot lighter physically, mentally and emotionally! Yanni informed me that over the weekend and many hours after the session, she could still feel the tremor tingling sensation in her legs. Her renewed energy was still moving up her thigh and down to her kneecaps! She told me that she was not expecting to experience all of this!

Many months later, I heard from Yanni. She told me that she had FINALLY tendered her resignation and did not retract it. She landed a new job with better package and happily moved on!

Finally, she found the TIME and the energy to pursue her passion. With a 'light' heart, she could revive her interest in championing a long over-due course which she believed in supporting and bringing local artisans with original ideas and empowering them to promote these ideas through her online platform. This is a platform that builds on community and sustainability to connect small, independent businesses to provide a genuine contribution back to the local community. Shortly after, she shared about another happy event that she is on the invited list to speak to groups of women about empowerment. She has also recently completed her long awaited degree on Childhood Studies and Counselling.

I celebrate with gratitude for this happy outcome. Yanni and her family so very much deserve it!

What I have learnt:

The 'harmony' that our body is in can be strongly influenced by emotional state, which in turn is impacted by cumulative recurring events around us. Similarly, like our immune system, our energetic fields can be misaligned over time. Likewise, our energy levels can be sapped by our attitudes and limiting beliefs. When there is disharmony, "everything" goes out of sync. Internally, when our thoughts, actions and feelings are out of balance, it can manifest at the physical level and give rise to serious problems with no clear medical solutions.

It is rewarding and enlightening to note that with JSJ, how powerful and transformative it can bring about for one who is open to healing. I am even more excited now that I have witnessed how this dynamic and highly intuitive ART can trigger neurological and physiological involuntary tremors leading to a release of deep tension, stress and trauma, restoring the internal harmony and recalibrating one's state of being!

Case 12 – Power of JSJ – boost speedy recovery

Caren works as a nurse in a private clinic. In July 2019, when she was at her workplace, she felt an excruciating pain in her lower abdominal area. She was rushed to hospital and had an emergency surgery done. The doctor had diagnosed the pain to be coming from multiple fibroids as well as a cyst in her womb. They were all removed and it was found that the largest fibroid was 18 cm and the smallest was 16 cm in size. Altogether, they weighed about 3 kg! It was her second fibroid related surgery. A surgery had been done 10 years earlier. This second time round, due to the unusual size and the state of her condition, Caren was advised to remove her uterus and ovary too. In addition, a part of her small intestine was also removed due to infection. The surgery took almost 5hrs and it was a traumatic episode in her life.

Post surgery, Caren shared that it was the darkest and the most challenging period in her life. Being away from her homeland, she felt very alone and miserable during this period of her life. Physically and mentally vulnerable. Caren was overwhelmed with feelings of helplessness as she could no longer carry out her daily routines independently. She had to rely on her husband and her mother, who came from the Philippines, to help with all her sleeping and waking routines. All day long since discharge, she could only lay flat on her bed as her energy was always depleted despite resting for the past weeks. Neither could she sit up nor go for a walk. Despite being as exhausted as an ox, she could not fall asleep easily. It was like having her body filled with wet sand and every part of her feels heavy and extremely hard to move.

Despite feeling flat like an empty battery, her body was too weak to even fall asleep! Her constant 'companions' were nightmares that further drained away her last ounce of vitality and strength. Due to the side effects of the anesthesia from surgery, she was also experiencing scary hallucinations which further caused her to keep awake so as to avoid the scary sight whenever she closed her eyes to rest. This soon took a toll on her speed of recovery and her mental-emotional state. With a heavy and weary spirit, recovery seemed elusive. She had to face a much longer recovery time and was given about 44 days of medical leave to recuperate.

We had the first JSJ session two weeks after the surgery. Caren was too exhausted to expect anything. However, she was very open and positive about the therapy. As the session continued, she shared that she felt something was going on. A calm and warm sensation began to circulate inside her body and the feeling seemed to envelope her body. She could not fully explain the sensation but soon this experience she said, "seemed to melt away my tension and made me feel so relaxed". Immediately after the first session, Caren was smiling because she bemused that "the feeling of heaviness on my whole body seemed to have gone." Physically and mentally she felt lighter and at ease. The next morning, I received a text message from her stating that she had slept well for the first time since the surgery. That night, she had slept soundly and peacefully without disruptions for a straight five hours. Her scary nightmares too seemed to have dissipated!

The next two JSJ sessions brought another level of recovery and relief for Caren. Caren and her family were very encouraged and thrilled with the outcome of the JSJ therapy. Not only was she looking more radiant, she was able to get up from bed *all by herself* and care for her own personal chores such as showering and going to the toilet independently. For the first time, her appetite improved tremendously. She could sit up straight for 2 hours at a stretch and take a slow walk around the estate where she lived at for some morning sun and exercise. The feeling of "emptiness" in her tummy was gone and she was able to move freely without pain. To further support and maximise the cumulative effects of the session, Caren was very diligent in the self-help homework I shared with her. Caren and her family could see the great progress since surgery. Each session seemed to boost her recovery rate. Although she was given 44 days of medical leave, Caren has fully recovered and reported back to work *3 weeks earlier* than expected! Thank you JSJ!

Case 13 – Restoring my TRUE self

Penny hails from overseas and whenever she flies down to Singapore, we would have regular JSJ sessions. We met in 2019 for weekly sessions and this has carried on since.

She is a qualified experienced masseuse and a Certified Human Design coach. Penny had also attended courses on JSJ. Amazingly, Penny has a special gift! She has a super sensitive body that can pick up energies within her body and from the environment.

Despite being in an endearing relationship for decades, Penny had neglected the needs of her own true self that needed nurturing. This neglect was attributed partly to the cumulative challenges in her relationship over the years. As much as she tried to fit in and please others in order to keep the relationship going, Penny was moving further and further away from being her true self. Being alone and away from home half of the time and having to face such mental challenges in a foreign land, was the last straw for Penny. Burdened with the constant state of roller coaster rides of emotions, she felt exhausted inside. She no longer delighted herself in her healing work as earlier.

To quote her, she said, "I was in an awful space and I did not want it anymore. I became so sick of it! I know the choice of a partner and the situation I was in wasn't great. I knew I had to stand up for myself because I just had to!" She continued, "I did not do anything wrong and I knew I did not want to be like that anymore."

Over the years, Penny met with many life-threatening accidents. As a result, she suffered constant tension and severe pain in her neck and shoulders which rendered her a little immobile as she had great difficulty moving and rotating her neck freely. Her lower limbs were also giving her problems making walking movement painful. She often had chest and respiratory issues too.

At the age of 36 years, she had had a hysterectomy and the doctor had accidentally cut her bladder! In that same year, she had her gallbladder removed and thereafter, unfortunately she suffered three major organ failures which included her heart, lung and liver ! Thankfully, she survived that ordeal.

At 39 and 40 years of age, she had a car accident where she had hurt her neck, shoulders, in between her left and right eye area, and her coccyx respectively.

She felt like she was reaping the effects of all her past 'traumas'. She fully understood that not living authentically subjects her body, mind, and emotions to unnecessary stress because her true nature was abandoned. Getting to know her True self takes courage. Penny fully understood that she needed an overhaul i.e. mentally, emotionally and physically.

Penny shared that she found JSJ as a timely and excellent tool which helped her unload layer by layer- mind body spirit level.

Time spent on JSJ sessions with Penny was most rewarding for both of us. We learnt from each other as we discussed the flows and how it affected her. During each session, Penny would experience different sensations within her body. She could even trace the path of the energy going through her body, sensing that 'innate' energy drilling through some obstructive areas in her joints. The pain seemed to move out through her toes and fingernails. As each session of therapy cleared and "tore down" what was needed for healing, she moved closer to harmony. She described it as "feeling alive again! It feels like "spring"."

Penny confessed that despite having a high threshold level for pain, there were times during the JSJ sessions when she felt like screaming the whole place down as the pain was intensely excruciating and unbearable. There were moments where she felt complete pins and needles on her whole arm followed by a heavy ache. It seemed like heat was coming out from her shoulders. She shared that the energy moved through her tissues and penetrated at the right spot. The areas in which she had borne the pain for years felt sore but relieved. It is interesting to note how the energy had moved through and healed all her past injuries or wounds that she had sustained. With regular sessions and diligent self-help, it was very encouraging to hear what she had to share-

"The sensation on my left shoulder (which felt like it was 'bulky') and the sensation on my chest seemed to have subsided...it seemed like all the 'puffed up' anger and frustrations had gone away. I came in with a very 'full and heavy chest' and what seemed like many layers on my neck. After a few sessions, I can see the contour of my neck and jaw line and no longer have a 'double thick chin'. I used to get very bad sciatic pain along my legs and hence I couldn't walk that much. I really felt lighter after each JSJ session with Nicole and I have also started going for long walks. I also felt an inner strength to stand up for myself and I spoke up for the first time in front of them!"

I have enjoyed the sessions with Penny as she is one of my few clients who has had an amazing feel for her 'sensing' body. We have both learnt much from each other and Penny continues to update me on how her self-help healing poses aid her in maintaining and harmonising her state of being. More importantly, Penny has regained her confidence and knows that she has the power to change and heal her situation and rekindle her passion in her healing work in JSJ and as a Human Design coach. Thank you Penny!

Case 14 – Bye Bye thyroid imbalance!

When I first met Tina in 2019, what caught my attention was her really skinny frame. It looked like even a light breeze would blow her off. Tina has lovely big bright eyes and a beautiful spirit.

She had emailed me formally for a session citing that her Reiki master had recommended JSJ therapy after she had tried many numerous but fruitless therapies for her serious condition. Besides the traditional medication, she has sought functional medicine to address her 'leaky gut' condition but without much progress.

Five to six years earlier, at the age of 49, Tina was diagnosed with autoimmune syndrome with pemphigus, a rare skin disorder that causes her skin to burst out in blisters uncontrollably. Three years later, she underwent D & C surgery to remove some polyps and fibroids. She also developed Grave's disease which is an autoimmune disorder that causes hyperthyroidism, causing a big swell at her neck area. With all these conditions, her immune system was also compromised. In addition, Tina had a 'leaky gut' syndrome that left her highly sensitive to a number of foods which she had to eliminate from her already limited diet. Some symptoms include fatigue, digestive problems, joint aches and pains, painful blisters over specific areas, insomnia and anxiety! To treat all these, she was placed on high doses of steroids for about six years, which led to her losing the ability to taste a year ago. Emotionally, she held a lot of baggage which often weighed her down.

During the initial sessions, she tended to be rather highly self-critical and hard on herself. She was very pessimistic about her slow progress. Tina was hoping to reduce the doses of steroids and have sufficient energy for her daily functions and hoped to eventually return to her work life and live a functional life.

Sessions with Tina were always refreshing because she would come prepared with notes and questions. She would diligently write down what she needed to do as her follow up (self-help homework) and she would return with even more questions at the next sessions. Even though she was new to this therapy and had not attended any formal training, she was very open and 'hungry' to learn to help herself. She has been one of the most hardworking clients I have had who would diligently read up and spend time doing self-help steps I shared.

It was very heartening to see her being transformed slowly but surely through the sessions.

Tina shared the following:

"The second session with Nicole somewhat magically brought an emotional shift which left me feeling positive and lighter. I had a great feeling which I had not experienced for ages. I realised I was trapped in the frustrating cycle of 'chasing' after my health against all odds. I always had dreams where I'd be in a maze going round in circles, holding the key to the solution but just not being able to get out of it. These recurrent dreams often lead to panic attacks and anxiety which trap me further. The process of doing self – help poses which Nicole shared with me and the JSJ sessions with Nicole somehow awakened my consciousness or awareness of my being. I also began to realise how my 'high anxiety' nature contributed greatly to my physical condition and state of being. After going through numerous thyroid tests and practising JSJ to treat it, the results showed improvement. I believe my body can heal itself too..."

On the 7th session, Tina shared that her thyroid tests had shown slight improvement. She also confessed and finally understood how her physical body would break out in severe skin rash all over her body due to her mental-emotional stress. It always deteriorated just before her blood test appointment.

On the 9th session, she shared that she could TASTE my homemade keto bread I baked for her. We were both so grateful for this to happen! Having to eat plain food and soup for years due to her leaky gut syndrome was already so sad. To lose one of her senses was like living life without colours. It called for more celebration and I continued to share my homemade treats with Tina.

In Dec 2019, she shared some more good news that her thyroid test results have improved further, but added that 'it was still not in the optimal range yet'. However, for the first time, her doctor was going to reduce the steroid dosage! Come Jan 2020, she revealed over a whatsapp message that the third thyroid test she underwent, she had PASSED the test after battling years with it. Finally she could STOP the steroid medication. With all the good news she received, she found impetus and energy to attend an intensive buddhist darma retreat course she had signed up for. It required her to do physical prostrations, something which she could not even do months earlier as she had to constantly contend with severe aches and pains. Tina came for a visit in Oct 2020, sharing with me that she has made real good progress. I could see she has put on some good weight and her face glows with more radiance than before. That persistent ugly patch of eczema near her lower eyelid and above her eyebrow is almost invisible!

Although her progress took time, she seemed to grow in self awareness about the issues she faced. I knew Tina could overcome all her obstacles because she had such determination and focus in her pursuit for self-healing. Despite her own challenges, Tina still finds time and shows loving kindness through her volunteering at a senior home on a weekly basis bringing cheer and hope to others. Thank you Tina!

Case 15 – Re-ignite my spark for life

Sky was recommended to me by a doctor to try JSJ to support his healing journey after a major surgery.

At the age of 45, he was diagnosed with a blood disorder exhibiting excessive haemoglobin levels. He was given medication for his 'thick' blood and 'very active bone marrow'. He shared that he often experienced high temperatures from 5pm onwards. He would wake up in the night sweating profusely especially at these three areas – his head, chest and butt.

Ten years later, when he had an upper molar removal surgery, he bled profusely for seven days. Then, during his quarterly medical scan, the doctor discovered an 'enlarged' spleen. Two years later, at the age of 57, his MRI scan showed a cancer mass growing and a very low blood count. With limited choices, Sky had to remove his spleen and left kidney.

As a result of the major operation, he was constantly suffering from low energy and he felt very weak. He could neither focus on any work projects nor sit comfortably for long to do his regular 'Huang Di Nei Jing' meditation. He became very frustrated.

Minutes after we started the first JSJ session, he opened his eyes and asked me why I was pushing him out of the therapy bed. He felt his legs shaking within and thought that I was deliberately shaking him off the therapy bed! He was actually experiencing immense energies flowing within his body.

The next day, he messaged and shared that he felt good and could feel the 'sparks' re-igniting in his body during his usual meditation routine. He felt like the lower part of his body had generated some heat and he managed to meditate for about 40 minutes holding his fingers after the session!

By the third session, Sky was looking better. His complexion seemed brighter and he had more vitality overall. It is interesting to note that each therapy session is very unique to an individual. For Sky, he felt a series of pain and heat radiating from various parts of his body such as his arms, legs, knees, calves, fingers and toes. He often felt 'sparks' igniting at his left kidney area.

Together with traditional medical support, JSJ therapy complemented Sky in his continual search for recovery. Keep it up Sky!

Case 16 – JSJ our beauty harmoniser

Aunty May, a kind and loving lady in her 60s, had a sad past. She was referred to me for JSJ therapy through her daughter. When I first encountered her, what struck me was her distinctively unusual high cheekbones. They seemed to pull her eyes so unnaturally tightly towards the back of her head.

Aunty May's husband had passed on many years earlier, but she was still holding onto her grief and loss. During each session, she would unavoidably share about her past. She shared that since his passing away, she had not stopped crying or sobbing. As a result of this overwhelming grief and constant outpouring of tears, her eyes had developed a strange disorder where there was involuntary closure of the upper eyelids. Unfortunately, this disorder had gotten her into many accidents. One of which, while she was crossing the road she realised that both her upper eyelids had unexpectedly involuntarily shut! She could not open them!

To solve this problem of her eyelids disorder, Aunty May had sought help through botox treatments every few months to ensure her eyelids were 'held up'. That was the explanation for her extremely unnatural high cheekbones and tightly pulled eyelids.

To our pleasant surprise, after a few JSJ therapy sessions, it was heartening to hear from family members that her cheekbones were no longer as high as before. Not only has her facial expression became more natural looking, more importantly, she has moved on with her life, letting go of her grief and feeling more emotionally happier. Thank you JSJ for restoring her inner harmony and beauty.

Case 17 – 'Smoke detector and detox'

Jass, CEO of a famous fashion industry led a very hectic lifestyle of incessant overseas travelling round the year. As a result, we only managed to have a limited number of JSJ therapy sessions. It is interesting to note that during one of the sessions, our silence was broken by a gentle emission of a smell that was somewhat similar to a cigarette! There seemed to be the 'smell' of a smoker lingering around us. I was somewhat worried if I was imagining it. I did not want to be distracted and continued with the session without disturbing my client. However, the smell became stronger as we continued the session. I had to break the silence and asked if she was a smoker. Jass shared that only her husband was a smoker. In fact, he was a heavy smoker. She told me that he is such a heavy chained smoker that he smokes almost everywhere he is in...at home, in car and as long as he is awake! She claimed she was not a smoker.

From this case, I learned that JSJ therapy has the ability to facilitate ridding the harmful intoxication (in this case smoking) accumulated over the years from a passive- second hand smoker. Perhaps it would also apply to any other 'harmful' invasion in the body. This explained why we could smell the scent of cigarette smoke! It seemed like the healing energy in the body has to, in some instances, cleanse first before repair works can start. I learnt from the JSJ lectures that among three accumulations in our body, gaseous accumulation is the hardest to get rid-off as compared to solid and liquid accumulations. I was very THANKFUL to be able to witness that!

Case 18 – How I beat Bell's Palsy!

Just as I was happily being busy with JSJ therapy and seeing a variety of interesting cases, I was suddenly struck with a form of paralysis one day. It was May 2017...

Looking back, I realised I had experienced some strange sensations that day. There was a tingling of heaviness and uneasiness around the areas of my eyes and it lasted for two days before I found out I had Bell's Palsy. On that fateful morning, while brushing my teeth, I noticed I had great difficulty holding water in my mouth during gargling. Water kept leaking from the left side of my lips. My lips did not seem to 'obey' my thoughts. I felt a weakness on the left side of my face. On closer examination in the mirror, I realised paralysis on the left side of my face seemed to have set in!

I tried to smile but to no avail. I just could not move the left side of my face! To my horror, I witnessed the left side of my face, from my hairline to my chin, drooping. It seemed like gravity was at play and when I tried to force a smile or even a grin, I could not do it. I could not even shut my left eyelid completely! I tried relentlessly for two days to get my facial muscles moving but the 'insubordination' continued. It did not get any better, and my mind went berserk.

I continuously asked myself a series of questions...

Was I having a stroke?
Would my face ever recover?

All the "What if" questions were racing through my neurotic mind. Instead of being calm and collected, I was entertaining thoughts of FEAR to its fullest glory! I quickly googled for information before even consulting a doctor! To add more salt into the wound, I had remembered someone I knew with this condition. That person had not fully recovered for over a period of two years. The internet research that I had gathered too did not seem to indicate that any patient with this condition got better within the few years of the onset...

Finally, I decided to make my way to the doctor and the visit to the doctor was brief. The diagnosis was clearly Bell's Palsy. I was told that the only cure was through medication like...steroids. I obediently took the dosage as prescribed as I did not want the inflammation to deteriorate into something worse. However, within a short time from taking my first dosage, my stomach walls felt like they were being stretched and torn apart. I could not bear the strong side effect of the medication and I started to vomit non-stop. Despite this, I continued with the next dosage for the day and my body reacted in the same way. The uneasiness of the tummy and vomiting added another layer of despair. I wondered what to do. My body was rejecting the "so-called" medical remedy, and I wondered how I was going to get better and rid my body of the condition. How was I going to help myself?

My own inclination was always to do JSJ to help myself whenever I felt unwell. Internally, I was also lamenting in my heart to the Divine, "Why do I have to face this at this moment in my life when I am so busy with my work and other projects to consider?"

It is very interesting how the Divine Hand of God works in my life. Over the next three weeks, all my cases were 'put on hold'. They were either on leave due to overseas travels or some events and hence we could not have any sessions. I literally had all the time to spend with myself and with my own project-Bell's Palsy.

With such a blessing of time, I decided to do my own JSJ self-help practices. I did it round the clock, only to stop for breaks during my meal times. My immediate observation was that with the daily self-help poses, I could stomach the strong steroid without any more vomiting! My body could accept the strong medication and I could complete the whole course smoothly.

Initially for the first week, I did not feel any improvement, or sense any progress. I still experienced dry eyes as my left eyelid could only close half way when I was sleeping. To protect it from further drying, I used an eye-patch when sleeping. My smile was still half droopy on one side and liquid from the cup would still continue to leak out when I drank or sipped from a straw or cup. I really felt like one who had had a stroke, as it was only half of my face that was affected. I could now understand

and empathise a little more now with all those patients with more severe symptoms. I felt like how many of them would feel in such a frustrating and devastating state. With this little insight, I actually began to feel very thankful and blessed for having this condition at that moment in my life.

I felt very thankful and blessed because I had such great support from my family. They were very understanding and all of them were helping out with household chores and left NOTHING for me to worry about or to do for the next 3 weeks.

They left me with plenty of time to spend with JSJ and Bell's. This was my project for that moment in my life.

To combat my sporadic pessimistic tendency, I armed myself with these as I did my homework with JSJ-

- I saturated myself with healing music;
- I read uplifting messages to motivate myself to continue with my self-help;
- I visualised and felt each of my cells regenerating as I did my hands-on self-help;
- I reminded myself about the successful cases of healing which I had the privilege to witness;
- I thanked the Divine for the experiences and the lessons to be learnt.
- While I was religiously spending time with myself and JSJ-ing my Bell's, I found my own psyche shifting gradually from the feeling of drowning in despair to being flooded with feelings of inner peace despite my horrendous demeanour. I was slowly flooded by a heightened state of divine and special awareness replacing my despair. Then, I knew I would get well.

I also thought of starting a photo journal of my own progress as I was sure to be able to encourage myself and any others who might be in the same situation as I was.

By the second week, as I was doing my self-help routine, something happened! I felt a faint sensation somewhat like a weak electrical current running through my lower lips, radiating towards my left lower lip. I could also feel the same sensation going through my left eye lids! Feeling excited and encouraged, I know that I was slowly getting healed and I knew I was going to get better!

Despite the progress I was making, my mother was still very worried and insisted that I visit a TCM specialist she had meticulously searched for. She wanted me to try acupuncture at the start of the diagnosis but I had resisted. The reasons being, first, I didn't like needles being pricked into my face (earlier, I was not ready for it). Second, I *knew* JSJ would help me and I wanted to go through this unique experience with JSJ myself.

As my mother continued to urge me to go visit the acupuncturist, I decided to combine JSJ and acupuncture from the second week. Somehow, I knew and had confidence that it would speed up my recovery.

I had contracted Bell's on 22 May 2017. I 'completed' my project of Bell's on 11 June 2017. I took a total of 171 photos as part of my healing journal. I knew I had gained a lot more awareness in spirit. To this day, I know that JSJ is a powerful healing art that never disappoints. I have also come to this state of understanding where I do not allow myself to get stuck, believing that whatever "limits" I have in my practice today will continue into the future. I know that there is no need to be discouraged if I do not have immediate results. I know that I do not need to be disheartened, even if I have practised for a long time without achieving amazing results.

I work with my philosophy of... 'What works for me...'. I am thankful for the medication I took, the TCM and most of all, JSJ in this eventful journey of mine.

I am truly Grateful for this project. Although modern medical interventions often play a critical role in healing, we are ultimately the ones responsible for our own harmony in mind, body and spirit.

CHAPTER 5

Moving forward

My life has evolved since JSJ made its way into my path. I have personally gained so much from this ART. I grew up with a neurotic essence in younger days and would worry about everything else that would not happen. My only 'peaceful' existence then was living through the need for certainty and over reliance on set formulae. No doubt life was unknowingly yet inevitably effortful and strenuous. JSJ has indeed transformed my being. The first and the hardest lesson I learnt is to trust and let go of my fear of uncertainty.

My Deepest Gratitude goes to all predecessors of JSJ and all the esteemed JSJ teachers who had crossed my path and guided me. Despite JSJ appearing in my life in the year 1998, JSJ was not my first choice of modality of therapy to consider. However, the experiences, the opportunities and moments presented to me during my life episodes at that point in time has drawn me to this art. It is as if JSJ 'chose' me and hence it resonates deeply with me when my heart is open to have a go with it. Since then, my journey with JSJ has been *exciting* as it continues to expose my ignorance and with new cases it brings me new found wisdom. I am still a student of this beautiful art. Indeed "it is a lifetime study".

Hence, in the initial years, I dedicated part of my afternoons providing JSJ services after my morning part-time work as a psychologist. Through this journey, I am also extremely grateful to SK for introducing and guiding me in this beautiful ancient ART. I would like to thank all my JSJ teachers that I have encountered; each contributing to my growth in different ways. I genuinely have never stopped learning from all the cases that came to me as there is no limit to our growth in JSJ.

JSJ has opened my mind and awareness to the dynamic relationships between the invisible and visible. As what Mary had shared, L I F E is "Look Inside For Everything". I find JSJ teachings present me with new ideas, new possibilities and the tool to realise those possibilities. It is up to me to manifest and start getting my hands involved. I have realised that JSJ completes the way of Life as what Mary Burmeister said. I am now a full time certified JSJ practitioner.

I have transited gradually from chasing test certifications and qualifications to finding fulfilment through impactful work that make a difference in clients life. Not meaning to sound arrogant, to me-JSJ is my BEST toolbox, one that is robust and timeless. This perfect tool needs no norms update or upgrade unlike various psychometric tools that often come with limitations and constraints over time and generations. Based on my own experiences in the wide range of projects or cases it has supported and helped, this ART IS indeed a dynamic and effective tool to embrace and treasure. It is no longer an iffy art to me but a fulfilling healing modality. I am now a true convert! No matter what diagnosis the clients are presented, JSJ always has its own unique, customised transformative solutions for each of them. The outcome is always HARMONY. This is the most beautiful treatment method I have seen. Indeed, the ART of Jin Shin Jyutsu is physio-philosophy, physio-psychology, physio-physiology. I am not exaggerating as you have read in the cases presented so far. You do not have to believe everything that I shared too. The only request I have is be open, go and experience yourself. Be your own testimony.

Most importantly, I hope the sharings in this book inspire you to start believing that you do have the power to heal yourself. Together with the simple use of Jin Shin Jyutsu, you CAN further restore and enhance your state of being towards a more balanced and happy self. As for me, I have a lifelong journey with JSJ and may I continue to age with JSJ. May this sharing bring you abundant blessings of harmony – mind, body, spirit.

CHAPTER 6

Self Help to Self Care

Main Central Flow

One of the hallmarks of Jin Shin Jyutsu is the wide range of self-help sequences which we could apply on ourselves using our hands as "jumper cable" hence we can always help ourselves as a preventive measure. It serves also as effective first-aid emergency while waiting for medical help in certain remote situations. Because of its non-invasive nature, this gentle therapy assures us of a safe application as it does not interfere with other treatments.

Among the many self-help sequences, the Main Central Flow is one of the most dynamic flows which many of my clients including myself had experienced. Hence, as care givers who are on 24/7 shift caring for others and no time for ourselves, this flow serves to boost our daily life battery within and with consistent self-help, it has cumulative effects to revitalise, restore and renew our Life Force within us.

The Main Central Flow is an All-inclusive source of energy for our being. It is the foundational harmonising energy flow of our body. It descends the front of the body to the pubic area and then ascends through the spine, flowing in an oval shaped circulation. This energetic circulation sustains all of the bodily functions, maintaining complete balance. When this main central flow is free from all 'blockages', it keeps us in great harmony and recharges us by revitalising all of our body's all other flows. With the Main Central flow, our being is brought back to balance whenever the energy is "unbalanced" on either side of our body. Hence our Main Central flow connects us with the Source of Life.

It is essential that we must be in comfortable position when doing this flow on ourselves, be it lying down or seated. As each of our body and its state of our energy within is unique to ourselves, doing this flow may have different harmonising effects for different individuals. Do note it is possible that some of us might experience some sensations such as occasional tingling, warm, yawning, jerks, pain, stomach gurgling, flatulence and etc. All these signs are indications that your body is in the process of harmonising. I would encourage doing this flow daily, before you start your day and just before you end the night. Remember this is *not* a technique. This is an art and hence it requires you learning to let go of the constraint of time, your noisy mental chatters and learn to listen within. Have a go at it and persevere through.

MAIN CENTRAL FLOW

Hold each of these 7 steps until a rhythmic purse is felt, or for a few minutes.

Each of these steps can also be used individually to harmonise specific needs as listed.

Follow the hand placement of this routine. In any comfortable position – sitting, reclining or standing.

Step 1 – **Right** Fingers or right palm on top of the head, Left fingers between eyebrows. This hold can be used to: • Revitalise the deep body energy circulation • Harmonise the pineal and pituitary glands • Stimulate mental activity • Improve memory and clarity of the mind	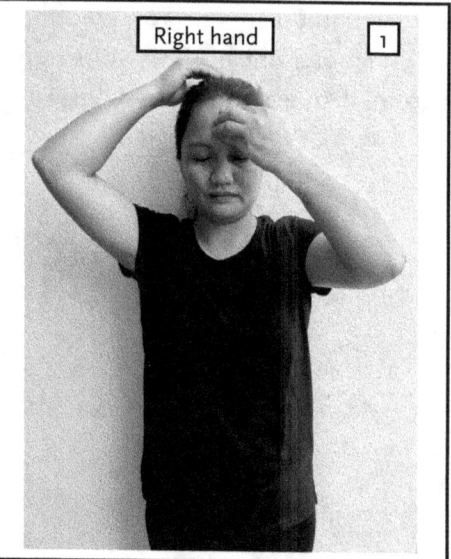Right hand 1

Step 2 – Move Left fingertips on the tip of the nose.

This hold can be used to:

- Energise circulatory system
- Release tension in the sinus
- Harmonise the hip areas and the reproductive functions

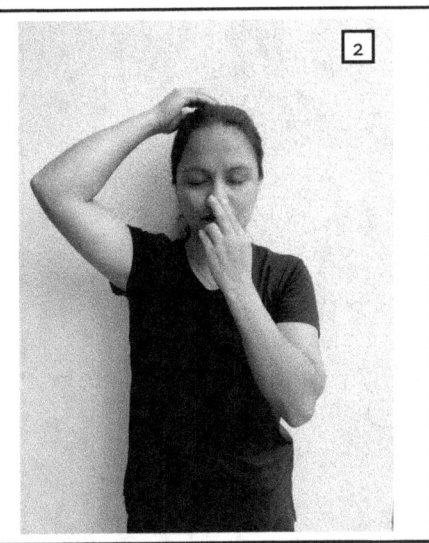

Step 3 – Move Left fingers to the hollow "V" of the neck-throat centre.

This hold can be used to:

- Energise thyroid and parathyroid glands
- Promotes facial muscles functions
- Find "your Voice"

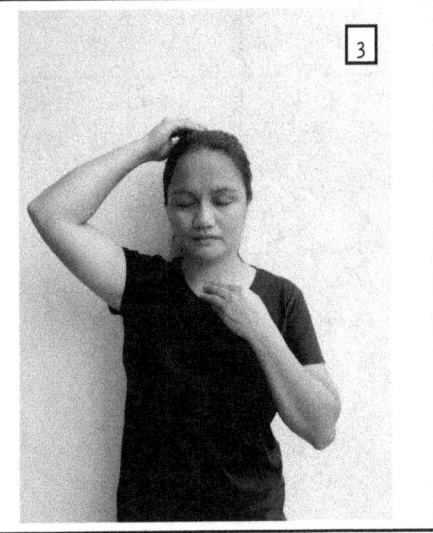

Step 4 – Move Left fingers to the centre of the breasts

This hold can be used to:

- Energise the immune system
- Revitalise energy for breathing and lungs
- Strengthen the circulatory system and pelvic girdle to support fertility
- Relieve nausea
- Harmonise our emotional balance

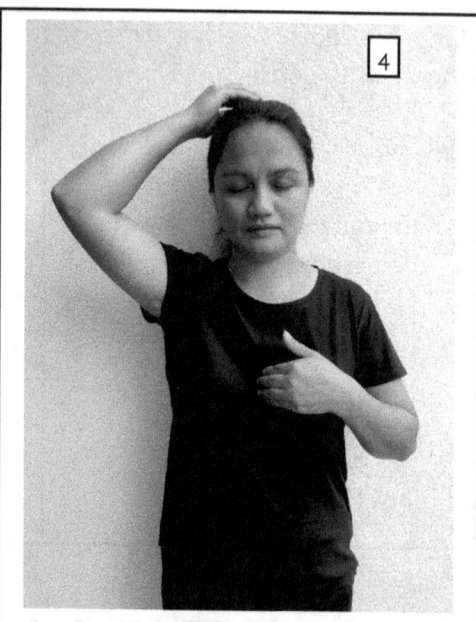

Step 5 – Move Left fingers to the base of sternum (around last rib, solar plexus)

This hold can be used to:

- Help both the descending and ascending energy
- Revitalise the Source of Life energy

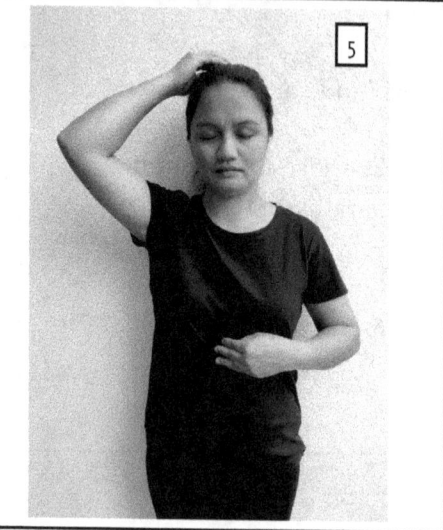

Step 6 – Move Left fingers to the top of the pubic bone.

This hold can be used to:

- Help energy to descend down the front of the body
- Strengthen the physical balance of the body and nourish spine

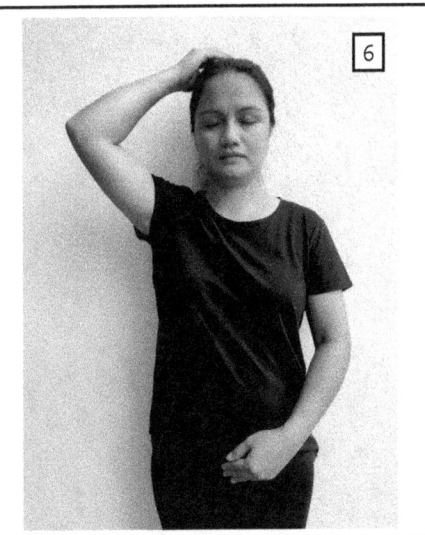

Step 7 – Move the Right hand to the tailbone (base of the spine)

This hold can be used to:

- Revitalises the rising energy of the Source of Life.
- Help the spine and circulation in the legs and feet.

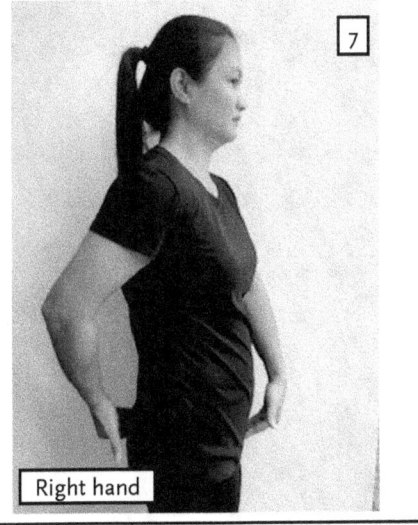

Right hand

ACKNOWLEDGEMENTS

With heartfelt thanks and immense gratitude, I would like to acknowledge the following amazing beings, who have made this book possible.

To all my clients who unreservedly shared how through the therapy of Jin Shin Jyutsu treatment had supported and transformed their darkest moments into incredible journeys of harmony and healing. Through your stories, you give hope and empower many lives.

To Jayanthi, my amazing editor, who asked for nothing but gave me the Best! You are one of my Divine Helpers who work tirelessly cleaning up my work! Thank you for giving your heart and soul into this creation.

My heartfelt thanks to Siew Kim for introducing me to Jin Shin Jyutsu. I thank the Divine for engineering you into my path during my early days as a psychologist in 1998 and how this beautiful ART has transformed my own journey as a user to a Jin Shin Jyutsu Practitioner. Thank you for all your precious time in those early days, guiding me and giving me opportunities to experience the magic of Jin Shin Jyutsu.

My journey as a JSJ practitioner would not be impactful without the generous sharing of knowledge and expertise from all the Jin Shin Jyutsu instructors from the Scottsdale Office.

Last but not least, I am immensely grateful to my family for their never-wavering support, belief, trust and willingness to be my first hand guinea pigs.

To my soul-mate and loving husband Joe, thank you for your unfailing support and encouragement to pursue this Magnificent Art. You had never doubted this from the very beginning, even though I was a sceptic then. Your intuition, patience and constant encouragement help mould my initial foundation journey with this Magnificent Art.

RECOMMENDED READING

Burmeister, Alice. The Touch of Healing. New York: Bantam Books, 1997.

Burmeister, Mary. What Mary Says: The Wisdom of Mary Burmeister. Audio edition. Scottsdale, AZ: Jin Shin Jyutsu, Inc., 1997

Riegger-Krause, Waltraud. Health Is in Your Hands: Jin Shin Jyutsu – Practising the Art of Self-Healing. New York: Upper West Side Philosophers, Inc., 2014

Glazewski, Andrew. Harmony of the Universe: The Science Behind Healing, Prayer and Spiritual Development. United Kingdom: White Crow Books, 2014

ABOUT THE AUTHOR

Nicole has more than 20 years of experience in the field of psychology and education, of which her first stint as a psychologist in 1996 began in the Singapore Prime Minister's Office and then the HQ in the Ministry of Education and the Special Schools. Nicole is considered to be the first psychologist trained in the Art of Jin Shin Jyutsu in Singapore. Her exciting journey with a wide range of families and individuals with learning, behavioural and special needs, sparked off her deep interest in the mysteries of nature and the psychology of mind and behaviour. This interest further fuelled her constant search for effective tools as remedy for those in need of harmony. Hence, her baby steps with Jin Shin Jyutsu study began in 1998.

She founded Hands Flow Pte. Ltd. (www.handsflow.com.sg), a company that offers a holistic approach for clients encompassing mental-emotional and behavioural intervention using the Art of Jin Shin Jyutsu. She works closely with all related specialists, therapists and case managers using a team approach to support the clients referred.

Since its conception in 2018, Nicole became the Psychologist Consultant for NannyPro, a "Business for Good" social enterprise that makes impactful contributions in the lives of homemakers and low-income families through life skills training. She spearheaded the Self Care Training Programmes which incorporates the Art of Jin Shin Jyutsu for the Onboarders and has trained many batches of nannies-to-be ladies.

Nicole resides in Singapore with her husband, who is also a psychologist and they have 2 lovely and harmonised teenage girls and a joyful pet.

www.ingramcontent.com/pod-product-compliance
Lightning Source LLC
Chambersburg PA
CBHW071025220526
45467CB00004B/1514